LOW-CARB DIET FOR TWO

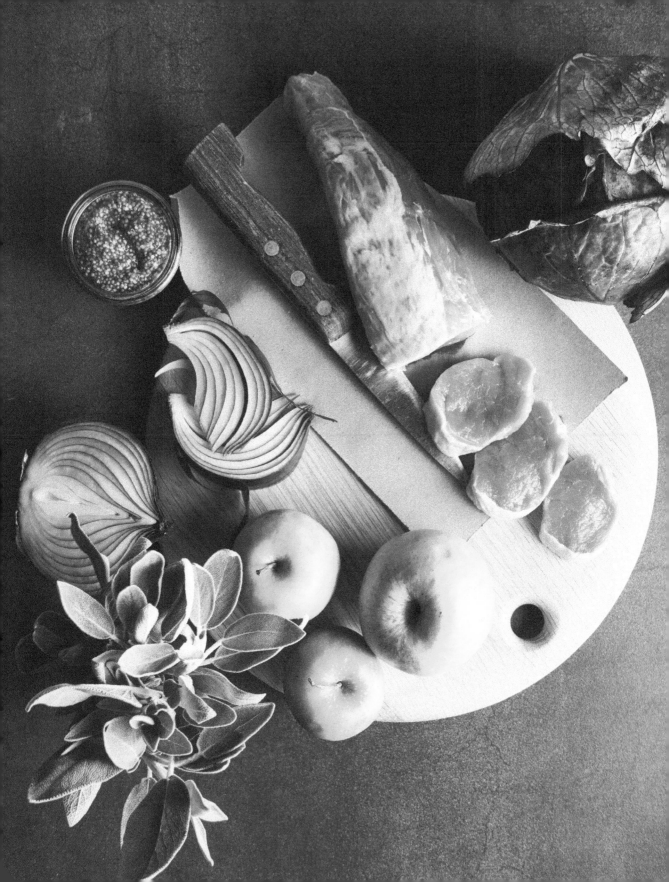

Bek Davis

LOW-CARB DIET
for Two

100 Easy, Flavorful Recipes
to Get Healthy Together

Photography by Marija Vidal

ROCKRIDGE
PRESS

For general information on our other products and services or to obtain technical support, please contact our Customer Care Department within the United States at (866) 744-2665, or outside the United States at (510) 253-0500.

Rockridge Press publishes its books in a variety of electronic and print formats. Some content that appears in print may not be available in electronic books, and vice versa.

Interior and Cover Designer: Jill Lee
Art Producer: Sue Bischoffberger
Editor: Ada Fung
Production Manager: Jose Olivera
Production Editor: Sigi Nacson

Photography © 2020 Marija Vidal. Food styling by Victoria Woollard.

ISBN: Print 978-1-64739-976-4 | Ebook 978-1-64739-977-1
R0

To Randy,
my husband and best friend.
We're a duo.

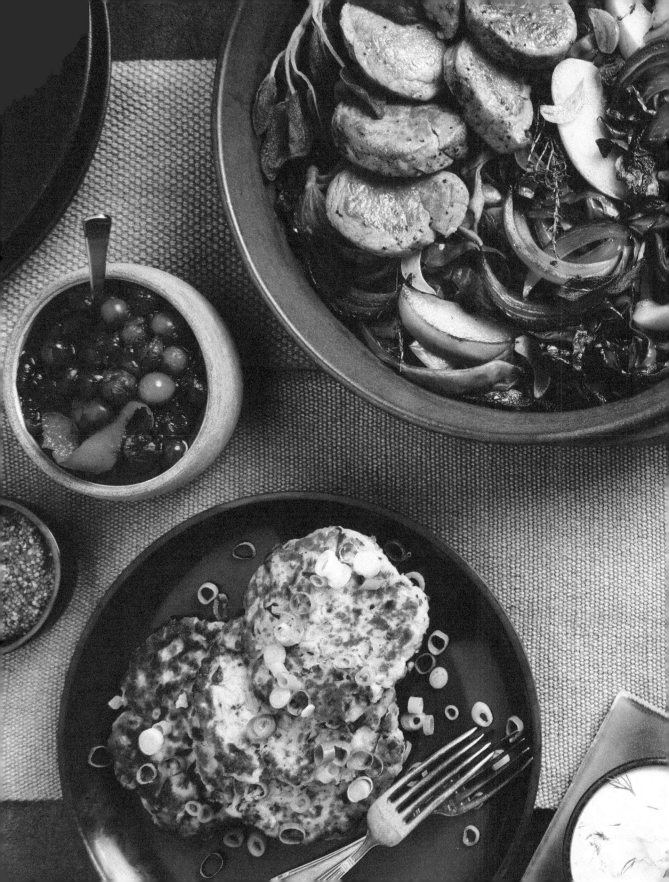

CONTENTS

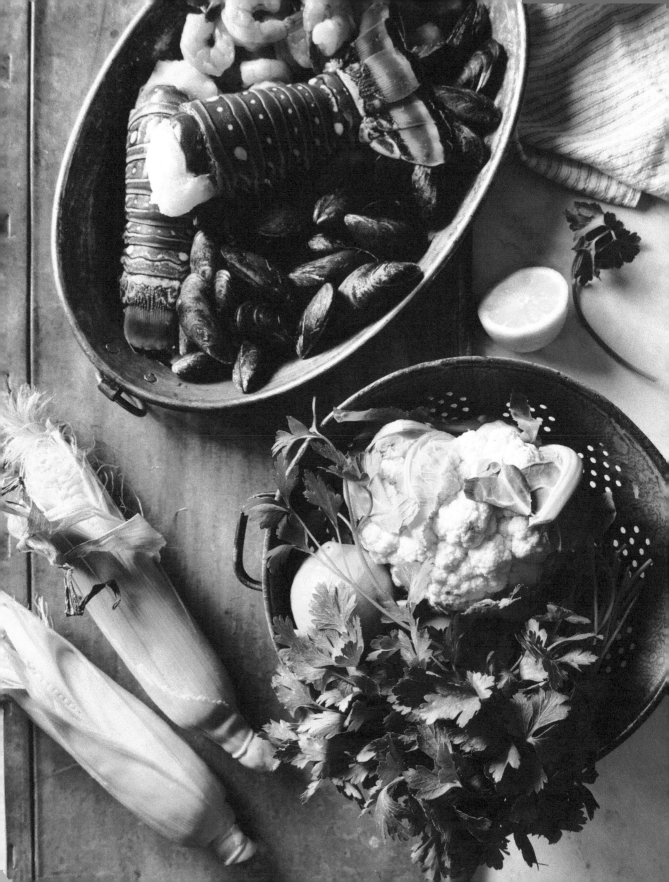

INTRODUCTION

I come from a large family of seven, and cooking and eating was always a major production in our home. I am the second oldest of five children, so I spent many hours prepping and cooking in the kitchen with my parents. Cooking quickly become a passion of mine at a very young age. I could always be found with my nose buried in one of Ma's cookbooks, skimming all the recipes, then running into the kitchen to check to see if we had all the ingredients necessary to prepare the dish. I later went on to formalize my passion of cooking by attending the Culinary Arts Institute of Louisiana.

After the birth of my second child, I found myself unhealthy, overweight, and miserable both physically and mentally. It was an eye-opening moment when I jumped onto the scale, staring at a number close to 200 on a 5-foot frame. I knew it was time to take charge and make some significant life-changing decisions. After many hours of research, I decided I was going to jump full force into adopting a low-carb lifestyle.

After a couple of weeks, the number on the scale began to drop and my body was feeling so much healthier. I could see my body physically transforming, my clothes were loose, and my mental state was in a much healthier place. The weight kept dropping and I was on a roll!

Our children have been cooking with me since they were babes, but they're now grown and have moved out, leaving me to learn to cook for just myself and my husband. Coming from a large foodie family and working in the culinary world, I definitely found this task challenging at first. I would find myself still trying to cook for an army, resulting in a surplus of leftovers that would go bad before we could get to them.

After some trial and error, I have learned that cooking healthy low-carb meals for two does not have to be expensive or result in leftovers for days. With this book, I will guide you through this low-carb cooking journey by offering shopping tips, meal planning tips, and 100 delicious low-carb recipes that will put you on the path to better health.

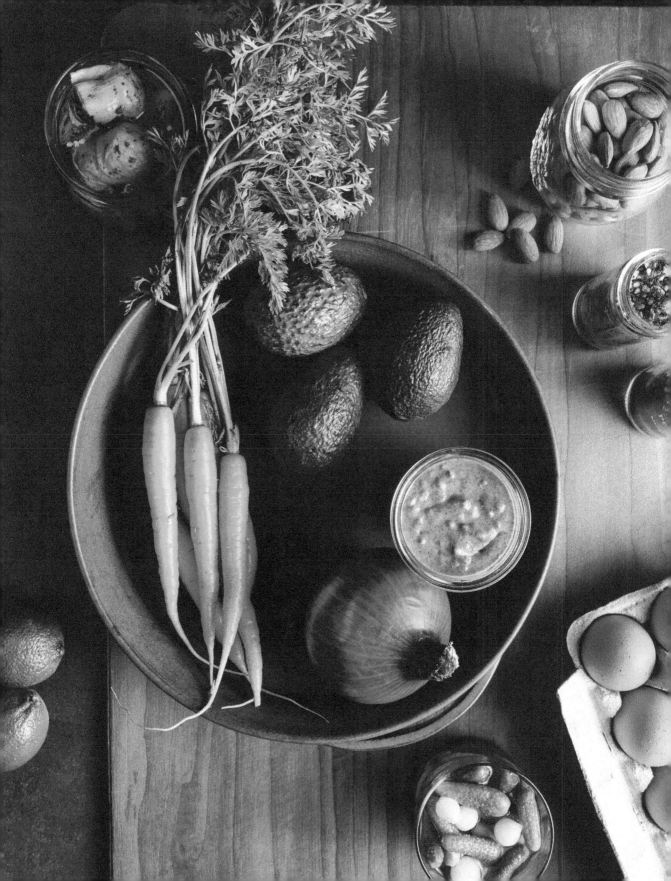

Chapter One

LIVING LOW CARB TOGETHER

Welcome to the amazing world of low-carb living! In this chapter, I will empower you to start eating healthier and give you all the information you'll need to jump-start your low-carb lifestyle. And because cooking smaller portions can be tricky when most supermarkets and cookbooks are designed with families of four in mind, I'll also be providing you with some useful tips for how to cook for two.

Low Carb 101

Before you dive right into your new low-carb lifestyle, there are a few topics that must be discussed. I will touch on exactly what carbs are, how they affect your body, and what it means to eat low-carb.

What Are Carbs and What Do They Do?

Carbohydrates are one of the three macronutrients, along with fat and protein. Macronutrients (macros) are the components of food that provide the body with energy. Carbohydrates are the primary source your body uses for energy. Protein helps the body build muscles and balance hormones. And fat helps the body absorb vitamins as well as keep the body feeling full for longer periods of time. All three macronutrients are required for your body to function at optimal levels on a daily basis. When you consume carbohydrates, your body begins to break them down into glucose, also known as blood sugar. Glucose is responsible for providing your body the necessary energy to function.

There are two types of carbohydrates, simple and complex. Complex carbs, aka "good" carbs, are those that are nutrient-rich and positively fuel the body. Examples of complex carbs are root vegetables, fresh fruits, legumes, nuts, and seeds. These "good" carbs are often filled with larger amounts of fiber and will help the body feel full for a longer period of time. Simple carbs, often referred to as "bad" carbs, are those that offer minimal nutritional value. Examples would be potatoes, rice, sugar, fruit juices, corn syrup, soda, and prepackaged sweet treats.

When "bad" carbs are overconsumed, it may result in an increase of blood sugar levels. This is because the body can digest these simple carbs more quickly than it can the more complex "good" carbs. For this reason, you may quickly feel hungry and tired. Consuming too many of these "bad" carbs can possibly lead to diabetes or other health issues. When reaching for carbohydrates, always steer toward a quality complex carb that will benefit your body.

If an excess of carbs is consumed, the body will eventually break them down and store them as fat. When you decrease your carb intake and "starve" the body of its preferred energy source, it must pull energy from another source. This is when fat steps up to the plate and becomes the new source of energy. Fat has twice as much energy as a carbohydrate (9 calories per gram of fat versus 4 calories per gram of carbohydrate) and will provide the body with more of a long-lasting source of energy. According to *Diabetes Forecast* magazine, when carbohydrates are scarce, the body runs mainly on fats. If energy needs exceed those provided by fats in the diet, the body must liquidate some of its fat tissue for energy.

What Does Eating Low-Carb Mean?

I am sure you have heard of, or possibly even tried, many of the popular low-carb diets out there, like keto, paleo, and Atkins.

This book falls under the "general low-carb" diet category, which means it does not adhere to any of these listed diets. However, many of the recipes will work for these popular diets, or the recipes can easily be tailored to meet the required macros of these diets. For this book, low-carb is defined as **80 to 100 grams of net carbs per day**. I wanted to give a range because there is a lot of variation in how people eat low-carb, and you should feel free to tinker and figure out what works for you and your health goals. So, you don't *have* to eat 100 grams of net carbs a day—you can stick to the lower end of the range, or go even lower if that works for you.

For your convenience when meal planning, I've made sure that the recipes do not exceed the following net carb counts per serving:

- **Breakfast:** 20 g

- **Entrée:** 30 g

- **Snacks, Sides, and Staples:** 15 g

- **Dessert:** 15 g

How to Count Carbs

Carb counting is imperative when following a low-carb diet in order to achieve success. The fiber in many whole foods is not fully digested by the body, so this is why we determine carb intake by calculating the net carbs. To find how many net carbs are in a product use the following formula: *net carbs = total carbs – fiber – sugar alcohols/sweetener (if applicable)*. The recipes in this book will give you the net carb counts as well as the macro percentages. Not everyone tracks these, but if you are on a keto diet, they will be useful to you.

Following a low-carb diet is wonderful because it allows for so much flexibility when meal planning. For example, you can plan for a lower carb lunch and dinner so you can enjoy that higher carb dessert or snack. You can decide what works best for you to stay under that 80 to 100 grams a day.

Comparing Popular Low-Carb Diets

DIET	NET CARB RANGES (GRAMS)	DESCRIPTION
General low-carb (*this book's diet*)	80 to 100	A moderately low-carb diet that focuses on whole foods and is less restrictive than other low-carb diets. It focuses on lean proteins, vegetables, fruits, and healthy fats. Some moderately starchy vegetables are occasionally consumed. This diet is more sustainable over the long term.
Keto	20 to 30	A very low-carb diet. The goal is to put the body into the state of ketosis to rapidly burn fat. This is a very strict diet with the macros ranging around: 70% fat, 25% protein, and 5% carbs.
Paleo	50 to 150	A low-carb diet that focuses on foods that come from hunting and gathering during the Paleolithic period. The paleo diet limits refined and processed foods, dairy, and sweeteners. Foods typically include lean meats, fish, vegetables, fruits, nuts, and seeds. Starchy fruits and vegetables are allowed on this diet.
Atkins	Plan 1: 20 Plan 2: 40 Plan 3: 100	A diet that offers three low-carb plans to meet the needs of the individual. Like keto, this diet also offers a plan that will force the body into the state of ketosis.

The Benefits of Eating Low-Carb

A low-carb diet offers many health benefits, and people turn to a low-carb diet for numerous reasons. Here are a few reasons to go low-carb:

To lose weight. When you restrict your carb intake, your body is forced to burn stored fat for energy. And replacing simple carbs with complex carbs (spinach, celery, kale, greens, and broccoli), lean protein, and fat will help you feel satiated over a longer period of time. If you're not as hungry, you'll find yourself eating less and naturally reducing your caloric intake.

To reduce your blood sugar. Decreasing the consumption of high-glycemic carbohydrates (pasta, potatoes, beans, rice, bread, etc.) will help reduce your blood sugar. Carbs increase blood glucose more than proteins and fats, so the body must produce more insulin to digest carbs.

To lower your risk of diabetes: A low-carb diet rich in healthy proteins and healthy fats helps in fighting, as well as preventing, diabetes. According to the Harvard School of Public Health, type 2 diabetes (as well as prediabetes) is largely preventable through healthy lifestyle practices, including controlling your weight, following a healthy diet, staying active, and not smoking.

To prevent heart disease: According to the Harvard School of Public Health, a moderately low-carbohydrate diet can help your heart health, as long as you're choosing healthy proteins and fats.

To lower cholesterol: A recent Stanford University study found that the group of low-carb dieters in the study who consumed a higher percent of saturated fats had better levels of blood lipids, including both higher HDLs (good cholesterol) and lower triglycerides, which are the main type of fat in the blood and in body fat storage.

Easy Low (and Lower) Carb Swaps

I thought it would be helpful to provide a visual chart of low-carb alternatives for some popular high-carb items. With a few simple swaps, you can begin to eat low-carb immediately!

HIGH-CARB ITEM*	SERVING SIZE	LOW-CARB SWAP	LOWER-CARB SWAP
White sandwich bread (14 g / serving)	1 piece	Low-carb tortilla (4 g / serving)	Lettuce leaf (0.1 g / serving)
White rice (22 g / serving)	1/2 cup	Brown rice (15 g / serving)	Riced cauliflower (2 g / serving)
Pasta (20 g / serving)	1/2 cup	Spaghetti squash (3.5 g / serving)	Zucchini noodles (1 g / serving)
Potato (12 g / serving)	1/2 cup	Acorn squash (6 g / serving)	Mashed cauliflower (2 g / serving)
Potato chips (14 g / serving)	1 ounce	Parsnip chips (4 g / serving)	Sliced cucumbers (0.9 g / serving)
Vanilla ice cream (15 g / serving)	1/2 cup	Frozen vanilla Greek yogurt (10 g / serving)	Vanilla Ice Cream, page 124 (2 g / per serving)
Milk (12 g / serving)	1 cup	Coconut milk (6 g / serving)	Unsweetened almond milk (1g / serving)
Most jarred marinaras (13 g / serving)	1/2 cup	Rao's Marinara (5 g / serving)	Classic Marinara Sauce, page 142 (4 g / per serving)
Premade pizza crust (17 g / serving)	1/2 crust	Light flatbread (12 g / serving) Low-carb flour tortilla (4 g / serving)	"Fathead" Pizza Crust, page 137 (2 g / per serving)

*All values are net carbs per serving.

Going Low Carb as a Pair

This is the exciting part, because we are about to dive into the logistics of going low carb together! I will walk you through how to purge your pantry and restock your kitchen with low-carb friendly foods. I will give you tips on grocery shopping for two as well as tips on meal prepping and meal planning as a duo. Ready, set, let's go!

Clean Out Your Pantry

The first step is to purge your panty of high-carb foods—out of sight, out of mind! Donate them to a shelter, family, friends, or neighbors. I've never met anyone who turned down free food! Get rid of:

- **Baking items:** sugar and white flour

- **Grains and legumes:** pasta, rice, breads, and beans

- **Snack foods:** crackers, chips, and pretzels

- **Sweet treats:** cakes, cookies, candy, and cereal

- **Sugary drinks:** soda, fruity drink powders, apple juice, pineapple juice, and cranberry juice

- **Sugar-loaded condiments:** ketchup, barbecue sauce, and teriyaki sauce

Although you will be doing this low-carb diet as a twosome, your carb restrictions may be different, or you may have others in the house who won't be eating low carb. If this is the case, I suggest having a designated area in the back of the pantry for the higher-carb items, so they are not front and center.

Shop Smart, Shop Small

Grocery shopping is one of my favorite pastimes. I've actually been known to call it a hobby. Having logged many hours at grocery stores, I have a few tips to help you shop smart for two.

Make a plan: Always have a game plan when going to the grocery store. Take some time to sit down to create a weekly menu. From this menu you can then create a shopping list. Having a plan tends to keep you from overbuying and adding unnecessary items to your shopping cart.

Shop the perimeter: The perimeter of the grocery store is where you'll find all the whole foods and healthy ingredients, so sticking to this area will stop you from impulsively picking up snack foods you don't need.

Except for the frozen and canned aisles: The frozen and canned aisles have great low-carb gems! Frozen and canned foods can be real lifesavers because they keep longer and cook quickly. But make sure you read the labels so you're not buying items with added sauces, sugars, or other fillers.

Say no to precut and packaged produce: It is a lot less expensive to purchase and prep fresh fruits and vegetables. For the precut, all you're paying for is the fancy packaging. Plus, precut veggies spoil faster.

Check the bulk bins: It might seem like contradictory advice, but the bulk bins can be your best friend when shopping for two. Here you can find nuts, seeds, nut flours, spices, dried herbs, and so much more, and you're able to scoop out and purchase only what you need for the week's recipes. This saves money and also keeps food waste down.

Visit the meat, deli, and seafood counters: Meat, seafood, and deli meats are typically packaged in large quantities. Many shoppers don't realize the same product can be found at the counters for the same price per pound.

Plan and Prep for Perfectly Portioned Meals

Just like any project or journey, planning is imperative for success and getting started on a low-carb diet is no different. Meal planning, portion control, and meal prepping will help you stay on track, minimize food waste, and set you up for success.

Sit down and write out a weekly menu: This will be your food and cooking roadmap for the entire week. Consistent menu planning will help you save money and keep food waste to a minimum.

Meal prep on nights or weekends: Meal prepping is a lifesaver when dieting. Prep raw vegetables and store in airtight containers for snacking and cooking. Precook some proteins to top salads or turn into lettuce wraps for speedy lunches. If you have the time, you can also prepare full meals and portion them out in individual airtight containers. Think of these to-go meals as your version of "fast food."

Plan multiple meals that use similar ingredients: Designing your menu around similar ingredients will save you money and reduce food waste. A leftover roasted chicken can be used in multiple ways: chicken salad, chicken lettuce tacos, chicken stir-fry, etc. I typically cook two to three meats throughout the week and plan my menu around those.

Inventory and purge: Look through your freezer, refrigerator, and pantry and plan a meal around what you currently have on hand. This will allow you the opportunity to use up any products that will expire soon and keep food waste down. This is great for the end-of-the-week meals. Get creative and make a low-carb soup or one-skillet bake from the week's remaining leftovers.

Be Each Other's Cheerleader

Jumping into a low-carb diet together can produce some amazing health benefits, and it can also be a wonderful bonding experience for the two of you. Here are a few ideas on how to be each other's biggest cheerleader:

Cook together: Spending time together in the kitchen will get both of you involved in every element of what goes onto your plates. You can learn from each other, develop a stronger bond, and create some new amazing low-carb dishes together.

Menu plan and grocery shop together: Make time to plan and prep your weekly menu together. This will ensure that you both have a say in what will be served for the upcoming week, and you'll both feel invested in the plan you made together. And the bonus is that shopping as a team means you'll knock it out twice as fast!

Challenge each other: A little friendly competition can be a way to motivate you to stay on track. Set a weekly weight loss challenge, a daily "steps taken" challenge, or a water chug challenge to get your daily water intake in. You can keep it fun and keep both of you focused on your goals.

Get moving together: Make it routine to take an after-dinner walk together, enroll in a class at your local gym, find a new-to-you hiking trail every week, or sign up for a local marathon together.

Encourage each other and ask for help: You're in this together! Sometimes your partner will need more help. And other times you'll be the one who needs a boost when the going gets tough. Ask for help when you need it, and if you see your partner flagging, lift their spirits by leaving handwritten motivational quotes on a piece of paper or taped to the mirror for your diet partner to see.

Your Low-Carb Kitchen for Two

I find that it's easier to stick to a diet when my kitchen is stocked with healthy staples. The ingredients listed here are used often in this cookbook. Hopefully you'll enjoy using them to chef up your own low-carb creations!

Pantry and Counter

- **Avocados:** I store ripe avocados on the counter, but I also like to keep a few unripe ones in the refrigerator, and put them out on the counter to ripen a couple of days prior to using them.

- **Baking products:** Baking powder, baking soda, extracts, and cocoa powder

- **Coconut cream**

- **Dried herbs:** Cayenne, paprika, chili powder, cumin, rosemary, oregano, and basil are some of my go-tos.

- **Flours:** I like to keep both almond and coconut flour on hand.

- **Low-sodium stocks and broths**

- **Nut butters:** Look for natural butters that do not have added sugar.

- **Oils:** Avocado, nut oils, olive

- **Sea salt and black peppercorns**

- **Sugar substitutes:** I use Lakanto Monkfruit—granulated, brown, and powdered.

- **Vinegars:** Balsamic, red wine, and apple cider

Refrigerator

- **Berries:** Blueberries, blackberries, raspberries, and strawberries

- **Butter**

- **Cheese:** I prefer to buy blocks of cheese to grate or shred because pre-shredded cheese has added fillers.

- **Citrus fruit:** I love to have lemons, limes, oranges, and grapefruits on hand to flavor dishes. I prefer keeping these in the refrigerator to extend their shelf life.

- **Eggs**

- **Fresh herbs:** Rosemary, parsley, cilantro, and dill are some of my favorites.

- **Fresh vegetables:** Broccoli, Brussels sprouts, cauliflower, mushrooms, and leafy greens like spinach, romaine, and kale

- **Garlic and onions:** I keep these in my refrigerator to extend their shelf life, but you can also keep them on the counter.

- **Heavy cream and half-and-half:** I use these products in my recipes because they have fewer carbs than milk. But if you're dairy-free you can also use nondairy milks, like almond or coconut.

- **Mayonnaise:** Look for full-fat mayonnaise. Avocado mayonnaise is lower in sodium than traditional mayonnaise.

- **Peppers:** Jalapeños, poblanos, and bell peppers are some of my favorites.

- **Yogurt:** Choose whole-milk low-carb plain or vanilla yogurt from Fage, Two Good, or YQ by Yoplait.

Freezer

- **Meat and poultry:** Pork steaks, beef filets, chuck steaks, turkey tenderloin, chicken breasts, and chicken thighs are always in my freezer.

- **Seafood:** Shrimp, scallops, salmon, cod, lobster tails, and tuna.

- **Frozen vegetables:** Riced cauliflower, spinach, green beans, broccoli, and shelled edamame.

- **Nuts:** Almonds, walnuts, and pecans are a few I like to keep on hand. I store nuts in the freezer because they stay fresh longer.

What's the Deal with Sugar Substitutes?

You already know that on a low-carb diet you'll be swapping sugar for a sugar substitute. But which one? Here are some of the popular substitutes currently on the market:

Erythritol sweetener: This is a zero-calorie, zero-carb sugar alcohol that does not affect insulin levels or blood sugars. Swerve is a popular erythritol blend that comes in granulated, powdered, and brown sugar form. The sugar to Swerve ratio is 1:1, making it easy to replace any needed sugar in a recipe. However, some have reported that it has a cooling taste when consumed in larger quantities.

Monkfruit sweetener: This is a natural sweetener derived from a plant grown in Southeast Asia and does not affect insulin levels or blood sugars. It also has zero calories and zero carbs. I use Lakanto, a popular monkfruit blend, in all my recipes. Lakanto comes in granulated, powdered, and brown sugar form, and it is also a 1:1 swap for sugar.

Stevia. This is a natural sweetener derived from *Stevia rebaudiana*, a plant from South America. It does not affect insulin levels or blood sugars, and also has zero calories and zero carbs. It is extremely sweet, so use in moderation, generally about half the amount called for in these recipes.

Kitchen Equipment

Here is a list of kitchen equipment necessary for creating the recipes in this book. I am sure you already have most of the items on this list.

Prep Tools

- **Blender or food processor**
- **Cutting boards:** one for prepping raw animal proteins and one for produce
- **Dry and liquid measuring cups and spoons**

- **Mixing bowls of different sizes**
- **Set of knives**

Baking and Cooking Equipment

- **3-quart saucepan**
- **10-inch nonstick skillet or sauté pan**
- **10-inch cast iron pan:** This is optional, but I love its ability to go straight from stove to oven.
- **Baking sheets**
- **Mini (3-by-5.75-inch) loaf pan:** I use these to make small-batch cakes and even casseroles.
- **Mini and standard muffin tins**
- **Slow cooker:** This is an optional piece of equipment, but I love mine! A 1½-quart one is great for two, but you can size up if you like to have lots of leftovers.
- **Waffle iron:** Optional, but I like the Dash mini waffle maker.

Low-Carb Recipes for Two

All these low-carb recipes have been created to serve two. However, there are a few exceptions for a handful of recipes that are well suited for leftovers, freezing, or just tasty treats to have around. I hope you find my recipes to be healthy, creative, and flavorful.

Recipe Labels

Each recipe will have the following dietary labels to assist in finding recipes that meet your specific needs: vegetarian, vegan, dairy-free, gluten-free, low-sodium (for dishes with 500 mg of sodium or less), and extra low-carb (10 net carbs or less).

Carb Counts and Nutritional Information

All recipes have a full panel of nutritional information, including calories, total carbs, net carbs, fiber, fat, protein, and sweetener. I have also included macro breakdowns, so if you're doing keto or if you just want to track your macros, you'll be able to do so easily.

Recipe Help

Each recipe in this book has one of the following tips:

Cooking Tip: Guidance for prepping and cooking the dish

Dietary Swap: Suggestions for swapping ingredients to transform the recipe into a vegetarian, vegan, dairy-free, lower sodium, or even lower-carb dish

Variation: Ideas for changing up the dish for a different take

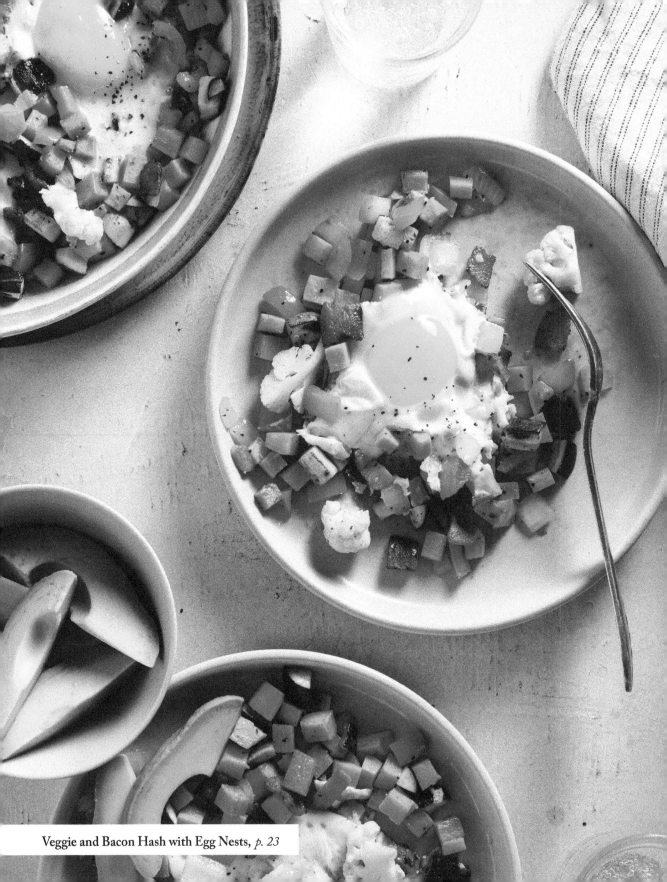

Veggie and Bacon Hash with Egg Nests, *p. 23*

BREAKFAST AND BRUNCH

Mixed-Berry Smoothies

Extra Low-Carb, Gluten-Free, Low-Sodium, Vegetarian
SERVES 2 | PREP TIME: 10 MINUTES

Smoothies are a convenient way to get in your daily fruits and vegetables—especially on busy mornings when time is of the essence—and this mixed-berry version is one of my go-tos. Using frozen fruit is super convenient, and it means you won't need to add ice to thicken the smoothie. Just make sure to check the ingredients of your frozen berries to ensure there is no added sugar.

2 cups unsweetened almond milk

2 cups baby spinach

1 cup low-carb whole-milk plain Greek yogurt

½ cup frozen mixed berries (raspberries, strawberries, and blueberries)

2 tablespoons granulated sugar substitute

1 teaspoon vanilla extract

½ teaspoon sea salt (optional)

In a blender, combine the almond milk, spinach, yogurt, berries, sugar substitute, vanilla, and salt (if using) and blend until smooth. Divide between two glasses.

VARIATIONS: For a peanut butter and jelly smoothie, add 2 tablespoons no-sugar-added natural peanut butter. Or, for a berry-chocolate version, add 1 tablespoon cocoa powder. Or leave the berries out for an even more versatile smoothie base that you can experiment with. Craving mint chocolate? Add some mint leaves, peppermint extract, and sugar-free chocolate chips and blend away!

Per serving: Calories: 130; Total fat: 6g; Saturated Fat: 3g; Total Carbs: 12g; Fiber: 3g; Net Carbs: 9g; Protein: 7g; Sodium: 150mg; Sweetener: 12g

Macros: Fat: 42%; Carbs: 37%; Protein: 21%

Apple and Almond Butter Parfaits

Gluten-Free, Low-Sodium, Vegetarian

SERVES 2 | PREP TIME: 10 MINUTES

Apples are nutritious and satisfying, and when paired with healthy fats and protein, they have a minimal effect on blood sugar and insulin levels. This healthy breakfast parfait with Greek yogurt, almond butter, almonds, and apple is a good option for people with diabetes who still crave something a little sweet to start the day.

1 cup low-carb whole-milk plain Greek yogurt

½ teaspoon ground cinnamon

½ teaspoon granulated sugar substitute (optional)

¼ cup no-sugar-added natural almond butter

½ medium red apple, cut into ¼-inch dice

2 tablespoons chopped almonds

1. In a small bowl, mix together the yogurt, cinnamon, and sugar substitute (if using). Spoon the yogurt into the bottom of 2 glasses.

2. Top the yogurt with the almond butter, apples, and almonds, and serve.

DIETARY SWAP: Lower the carbs in this recipe by using raspberries or cherries instead of the apple. Both pair well with almonds.

Per serving: Calories: 339; Total fat: 25g; Saturated Fat: 4g; Total Carbs: 21g; Fiber: 6g; Net Carbs: 15g; Protein: 12g; Sodium: 59mg; Sweetener: 0g

Macros: Fat: 62%; Carbs: 26%; Protein: 14%

Nut and Seed Granola
with Greek Yogurt

Extra Low-Carb, Gluten-Free, Low-Sodium, Vegetarian

MAKES 3½ CUPS GRANOLA | PREP TIME: 10 MINUTES | COOK TIME: 25 MINUTES

Granola and yogurt are perfect when you are in a hurry or looking for a lighter source of energy to jump-start your morning. I know, I know, this recipe makes more than two servings, but I love making this granola in bulk because it is so versatile. Add it to a salad or a cup of my Vanilla Ice Cream (page 124). The granola can be stored in an airtight container at room temperature for a week.

1 cup sliced almonds

1 cup chopped walnuts

1 cup chopped pecans

⅓ cup brown
  sugar substitute

¼ cup pumpkin seeds

¼ cup sunflower seeds

¼ cup unsweetened
  coconut flakes

¼ cup coconut oil, melted

1 large egg white

1 teaspoon vanilla extract

1 cup low-carb whole-milk
  plain Greek yogurt

1. Preheat the oven to 300°F. Line a baking sheet with parchment paper.

2. In a medium bowl, combine the almonds, walnuts, pecans, sugar substitute, pumpkin seeds, sunflower seeds, and coconut flakes and mix well.

3. In a small bowl, whisk together the oil, egg white, and vanilla. Add to the nut mixture and mix until well incorporated.

4. Evenly spread the mixture onto the prepared baking sheet. Bake for 20 to 25 minutes, until golden brown. Remove from the oven and let cool for 5 minutes. With a spatula, scrape the granola off the pan and break into smaller pieces.

5. To serve, divide the Greek yogurt between two bowls and top each with ½ cup granola.

Per serving (½ cup granola): Calories: 428; Total fat: 42g; Saturated Fat: 11g; Total Carbs: 9g; Fiber: 5g; Net Carbs: 4g; Protein: 10g; Sodium: 10mg; Sweetener: 9g

Macros: Fat: 83%; Carbs: 9%; Protein: 8%

Per serving (granola plus yogurt): Calories: 503; Total fat: 46g; Saturated Fat: 13g; Total Carbs: 15g; Fiber: 5g; Net Carbs: 10g; Protein: 14g; Sodium: 66mg; Sweetener: 9g

Macros: Fat: 78%; Carbs: 12%; Protein: 10%

Open-Faced Mediterranean Omelet

Gluten-Free

SERVES 2 | PREP TIME: 10 MINUTES | COOK TIME: 10 MINUTES

This protein-packed breakfast just bursts with flavor. The smoked salmon brings some amazing omega-3 fats to the dish, which is wonderful for the brain; the fat will also help keep you full longer. This dish is also ideal for a lunch or dinner on a lazy night.

1 tablespoon extra-virgin olive oil

4 large eggs, beaten

¼ teaspoon sea salt

¼ teaspoon freshly ground black pepper

1 cup chopped baby spinach

2 canned artichoke hearts, chopped

4 Greek olives, pitted and sliced

½ Roma (plum) tomato, sliced

¼ cup crumbled feta cheese

1 tablespoon chopped fresh dill, plus more for garnish

4 ounces smoked salmon, chopped

½ lemon

1. In medium skillet, heat the oil over medium-high heat for about 30 seconds.

2. In a small bowl, season the eggs with the salt and pepper and pour into the skillet. Swirl to coat the bottom of the skillet with the eggs and cook for about 5 minutes, or until the eggs are set.

3. Reduce the heat to low and top the eggs with the spinach, artichoke hearts, olives, tomato, feta, and dill. Cover and cook for 5 minutes, or until the cheese begins to soften and the spinach wilts. Remove from the heat.

4. Evenly distribute the salmon on top of the omelet.

5. To serve, cut the omelet in half and garnish with additional dill and a squeeze of lemon juice.

DIETARY SWAP: Lower the calories, fat, and cholesterol by replacing the whole eggs with 8 egg whites.

Per serving: Calories: 405; Total fat: 24g; Saturated Fat: 8g; Total Carbs: 19g; Fiber: 8g; Net Carbs: 11g; Protein: 31g; Sodium: 1,565mg; Sweetener: 0g

Macros: Fat: 53%; Carbs: 16%; Protein: 31%

Egg, Spinach, and Gouda Stuffed Portobello Mushrooms

Extra Low-Carb, Gluten-Free, Vegetarian

SERVES 2 | PREP TIME: 10 MINUTES | COOK TIME: 20 MINUTES

Portobello mushrooms are a game-changer when living a low-carb lifestyle. I stuff portobellos with so many delicious combinations, but this rich and creamy breakfast version is one of my favorites. Serve these mushrooms over a bed of mixed greens for a heartier meal and additional nutrition.

4 large portobello mushroom caps, stems removed and gills scraped out

1 teaspoon sea salt

1 teaspoon freshly ground black pepper

1 cup chopped baby spinach

4 large eggs

½ cup shredded Gouda cheese

1. Preheat the oven to 350°F. Line a baking sheet with parchment paper.

2. Set the mushrooms on the prepared baking sheet, stemmed-side up, and season with the salt and pepper. Dividing evenly, top the mushrooms with the spinach.

3. Into a small bowl, crack 1 egg at a time, and carefully spoon each onto the top of the spinach. Top each mushroom with 2 tablespoons of Gouda.

4. Bake for 15 to 20 minutes, until the egg whites are fully cooked or the desired doneness is achieved.

COOKING TIP: After removing the stems from the mushrooms, use a spoon to scrape out the black gills to make room for the filling.

Per serving: Calories: 289; Total fat: 19g; Saturated Fat: 9g; Total Carbs: 8g; Fiber: 3g; Net Carbs: 5g; Protein: 23g; Sodium: 1,416mg; Sweetener: 0g

Macros: Fat: 58%; Carbs: 10%; Protein: 32%

Veggie and Bacon Hash with Egg Nests

Dairy-Free, Gluten-Free

SERVES 2 | PREP TIME: 10 MINUTES | COOK TIME: 25 MINUTES

I like to prepare this brunch dish on a late Saturday morning for my husband and me. The combination of bacon, onion, sweet potatoes, and smoked paprika just can't be beat. I have a feeling this one will become a weekend brunch tradition for you, too.

2 bacon slices, chopped

½ head cauliflower, cut into ¼-inch dice

½ zucchini, cut into ½-inch cubes

½ white onion, chopped

½ red bell pepper, cut into ½-inch squares

⅓ cup sweet potato, cut into ¼-inch dice

½ teaspoon smoked paprika

½ teaspoon sea salt

½ teaspoon freshly ground black pepper

4 large eggs

1 avocado, sliced

1. In a medium skillet, cook the bacon over medium heat for 6 to 8 minutes, until slightly crispy. Remove from the pan and place on a plate lined with paper towels.

2. Add the cauliflower, zucchini, onion, bell pepper, sweet potato, smoked paprika, salt, and black pepper. Cook for 8 to 10 minutes, stirring occasionally, until the vegetables become tender and golden. Return the bacon to the pan.

3. Make 4 holes in the hash and crack an egg into each hole. Cover and cook for 5 minutes, or until your desired doneness of the egg is reached.

4. Divide evenly between two plates and garnish with avocado slices.

DIETARY SWAP: Make this vegetarian by omitting the bacon or substituting extra-firm tofu. This will also reduce the fat and sodium levels.

Per serving: Calories: 435; Total fat: 29g; Saturated Fat: 7g; Total Carbs: 27g; Fiber: 12g; Net Carbs: 15g; Protein: 22g; Sodium: 939mg; Sweetener: 0g

Macros: Fat: 57%; Carbs: 23%; Protein: 20%

Drop Biscuits with Onion and Mushroom Gravy

Gluten-Free, Vegetarian

SERVES 2 | PREP TIME: 10 MINUTES | COOK TIME: 30 MINUTES

This special-occasion breakfast is so rich and flavorful it will have you questioning whether it is low-carb. These biscuits can also be eaten alongside a soup or salad, or turned into garlic bread. Don't hesitate to double this biscuit recipe to have extras on hand!

2 tablespoons almond flour

2 tablespoons coconut flour

¾ teaspoon baking powder

½ teaspoon sea salt, divided

2 tablespoons sour cream

1 large egg

1 tablespoon butter, melted

2 tablespoons extra-virgin olive oil

2 cups sliced white mushrooms

½ white onion, chopped

¼ teaspoon freshly ground black pepper

1 cup heavy (whipping) cream

1. Preheat the oven to 350°F. Line a baking sheet with parchment paper.

2. In a large bowl, mix the almond flour, coconut flour, baking powder, and ¼ teaspoon of salt. Add the sour cream, egg, and melted butter and mix well.

3. Evenly spoon the batter onto the prepared baking sheet, making 6 evenly sized biscuits. Bake for 20 to 25 minutes, until browned.

4. Meanwhile, in a medium skillet, heat the oil over medium-high heat. Add the mushrooms and onion and cook for 7 to 9 minutes, until the vegetables begin to brown. Season with the remaining ¼ teaspoon of salt and the pepper.

5. Reduce the heat to medium-low and add the cream. Cook for 5 minutes, stirring frequently to deglaze the skillet and scrape up the browned bits from the bottom, until the sauce reduces and thickens. The end result should slightly coat the back of a spoon.

6. Split the biscuits in half horizontally. Arrange 3 halved biscuits each on two plates. Dividing evenly, slather them with mushroom gravy and serve hot.

VARIATION: To make a sausage gravy, add 8 ounces of breakfast sausage after you sauté the mushrooms and onion, but make sure to drain any excess grease before adding the heavy cream.

Per serving: Calories: 705; Total fat: 70g; Saturated Fat: 0g; Total Carbs: 15g; Fiber: 4g; Net Carbs: 11g; Protein: 10g; Sodium: 604mg; Sweetener: 0g

Macros: Fat: 90%; Carbs: 5%; Protein: 5%

Prosciutto Vegetable Egg Cups

Extra Low-Carb, Gluten-Free

SERVES 2 | PREP TIME: 10 MINUTES | COOK TIME: 20 MINUTES

I like to make a bigger batch of these delicious breakfast bombs on weekends to store in the refrigerator for those busy weekday mornings. They are super convenient to heat up and even eat on the go! The vegetable combinations of this recipe are limitless—play with your favorite veggie combos and make this recipe uniquely yours.

Extra-virgin olive oil, for greasing

4 prosciutto slices

½ cup shredded mozzarella cheese

¼ cup heavy (whipping) cream

½ Roma (plum) tomato, diced

2 large eggs

¼ green bell pepper, diced

1 tablespoon chopped scallions, green tops only

2 to 3 fresh basil leaves, chopped

¼ teaspoon sea salt

½ teaspoon freshly ground black pepper

1. Preheat the oven to 375°F. Grease 4 cups of a standard muffin tin with oil.

2. Line each cup with one slice of prosciutto until fully covered, overlapping if necessary.

3. In a medium bowl, whisk together the mozzarella, cream, tomato, eggs, bell pepper, scallion greens, basil, salt, and black pepper. Evenly divide the egg batter among the cups.

4. Bake for 15 to 20 minutes, until the eggs are cooked throughout and golden. Cool for 5 minutes in the pan on a wire rack.

5. Set 2 egg cups each on two plates and serve warm.

COOKING TIP: These egg cups can also be prepared in a mini muffin tin to produce 8 cups. Bake them at the same temperature for 10 to 15 minutes.

Per serving: Calories: 330; Total fat: 27g; Saturated Fat: 13g; Total Carbs: 4g; Fiber: 1g; Net Carbs: 3g; Protein: 18g; Sodium: 670mg; Sweetener: 0g

Macros: Fat: 72%; Carbs: 5%; Protein: 23%

Smoked Salmon and Egg Breakfast Sandwiches

Extra Low-Carb, Gluten-Free

SERVES 2 | PREP TIME: 10 MINUTES | COOK TIME: 5 MINUTES

Breakfast sandwiches are always so convenient to add to your rotation. This smoked salmon version is my take on a smoked salmon bagel sandwich without all the carbs. It also makes a speedy lunch option.

3 large eggs
¼ teaspoon sea salt
¼ teaspoon freshly ground black pepper
½ tablespoon butter
4 ounces sliced smoked salmon

2 ounces full-fat cream cheese, cut into chunks
Double recipe (4 "slices") Soft and Fluffy Sandwich Bread (page 136)

1 cup mixed greens
½ avocado, sliced
4 cucumber slices

1. In a bowl, whisk together the eggs, salt, and pepper.

2. In a skillet, melt the butter over medium-low heat and cook for 30 seconds, until bubbling. Add the eggs to the pan and, using a silicone spatula, constantly stir until small curds form. Add the salmon and cream cheese and stir for an additional 30 to 45 seconds, until large curds are formed.

3. Assemble the sandwiches in the following order: 1 slice bread, mixed greens, avocado slices, cucumber slices, scrambled eggs, and second slice bread.

COOKING TIP: The key to a perfectly creamy soft-cooked egg is cooking over low heat and gently scraping the bottom of the pan to ensure there is no burning.

Per serving: Calories: 674; Total fat: 54g; Saturated Fat: 16g; Total Carbs: 13g; Fiber: 7g; Net Carbs: 6g; Protein: 34g; Sodium: 2,097mg; Sweetener: 0g

Macros: Fat: 72%; Carbs: 8%; Protein: 20%

Vegetable and Brie Breakfast Casserole

Gluten-Free, Vegetarian

SERVES 2 | PREP TIME: 15 MINUTES | COOK TIME: 40 MINUTES

This loaded breakfast casserole is sure to please anyone. The key is to cook the veggies before combining them with the egg mixture to enhance the sweetness of the onions and the earthiness of the mushrooms and zucchini. I like to serve this dish sliced on a lightly dressed arugula salad.

Nonstick cooking spray

1 tablespoon extra-virgin olive oil

1 medium zucchini, cut into ¼-inch dice

½ white onion, chopped

½ red bell pepper, chopped

½ cup ¼-inch dice mushrooms

2 garlic cloves, minced

4 large eggs

½ cup half-and-half

½ tablespoon Dijon mustard

½ teaspoon sea salt

½ teaspoon freshly ground black pepper

1 cup chopped baby spinach

4 ounces Brie cheese, chopped (removing the rind is optional)

1. Preheat the oven to 350°F. Mist a mini loaf pan with cooking spray.

2. In a large skillet, heat the oil over medium-high heat. Add the zucchini, onion, bell pepper, mushrooms, and garlic and cook for 7 to 9 minutes, until the vegetables begin to soften. Allow to cool for 5 minutes.

3. In a large bowl, whisk together the eggs, half-and-half, mustard, salt, and black pepper. Mix in the spinach and Brie until well combined. Fold the cooled vegetable mixture into the egg mixture.

4. Pour into the prepared loaf pan, cover with aluminum foil, and bake for 25 to 30 minutes, until the egg custard is cooked through and firm.

5. Let sit for 5 minutes, then cut into slices to serve.

DIETARY SWAP: Replace the Dijon mustard with ¼ teaspoon mustard powder to reduce the sodium level.

Per serving: Calories: 426; Total fat: 40g; Saturated Fat: 18g; Total Carbs: 14g; Fiber: 3g; Net Carbs: 11g; Protein: 29g; Sodium: 1,055mg; Sweetener: 0g

Macros: Fat: 67%; Carbs: 10%; Protein: 23%

Pumpkin Pecan Waffles with Cinnamon Ricotta

Extra Low-Carb, Gluten-Free, Low-Sodium, Vegetarian

MAKES 4 MINI WAFFLES OR 2 STANDARD WAFFLES | PREP TIME: 10 MINUTES | COOK TIME: 10 MINUTES

I believe pumpkin season should be celebrated year-round! These tasty waffles are light and fluffy with the warm flavors of fall. The subtle sweetness of the Italian ricotta cheese complements the earthy pumpkin flavor quite nicely. This batter can be made into pancakes if you don't have a waffle maker.

½ cup almond flour

2 ounces full-fat cream cheese, at room temperature

2 large eggs

2½ tablespoons brown sugar substitute, divided

1 tablespoon unsweetened canned pumpkin puree (not pie filling)

2 teaspoons ground cinnamon

1 teaspoon baking powder

½ teaspoon ground nutmeg

⅛ teaspoon sea salt

2 tablespoons chopped pecans

½ cup ricotta cheese

1. Preheat a mini waffle iron or standard waffle iron according to the manufacturer's instructions.

2. In a blender, combine the almond flour, cream cheese, eggs, 2 tablespoons of brown sugar substitute, pumpkin, cinnamon, baking powder, nutmeg, and salt and process until smooth. Stir in the pecans.

3. Pour a scoop of the batter (according to the manufacturer's instructions) onto the waffle iron and cook until golden brown. Remove the waffle and repeat with the remaining batter.

4. In a small bowl, mix the ricotta and remaining ½ tablespoon of brown sugar substitute until well incorporated.

5. Serve 2 minis or 1 standard waffle per person, topped with the ricotta mixture.

DIETARY SWAP: If you're watching your sodium intake, use reduced sodium baking powder to reduce the sodium by almost half.

Per serving: Calories: 475; Total fat: 40g; Saturated Fat: 14g; Total Carbs: 29g; Fiber: 5g; Net Carbs: 9g; Protein: 21g; Sodium: 307mg; Sweetener: 15g

Macros: Fat: 72%; Carbs: 10%; Protein: 18%

Pecan French Toast in a Mug

Extra Low-Carb, Gluten-Free, Low-Sodium, Vegetarian

SERVES 2 | PREP TIME: 5 MINUTES | COOK TIME: 2 MINUTES

Mug cakes make cooking for two so much less time-consuming, and French toast has always been our weekend go-to. This recipe combines the ease of a mug cake with the decadent flavors of French toast to make a low-carb weekend brunch dish that will not disappoint. Swap out the vanilla extract for pumpkin pie extract for a warmer and more fall-like flavor.

Nonstick cooking spray

⅓ cup almond flour

1 tablespoon brown sugar substitute

2 teaspoons chopped pecans

¼ teaspoon ground cinnamon

¼ teaspoon sea salt

⅛ teaspoon ground nutmeg

2 large eggs

2 teaspoons unsweetened almond milk

2 teaspoons butter, melted

½ teaspoon vanilla extract

Sugar-free maple-flavored syrup, for serving (optional)

1. Mist 2 microwave-safe mugs with cooking spray.

2. In a small bowl, mix together the almond flour, brown sugar substitute, pecans, cinnamon, salt, and nutmeg.

3. Stir in the eggs, almond milk, melted butter, and vanilla until well incorporated.

4. Divide the batter evenly between the mugs. Microwave on high for 1 to 1½ minutes, until the batter is firm to the touch.

5. Serve warm with your favorite sugar-free maple-flavored syrup, if using.

COOKING TIP: Keep a close eye when cooking to prevent overcooking. Start by cooking for 1 minute and check to see if additional cooking time is necessary. All microwaves vary.

Per serving: Calories: 212; Total fat: 18g; Saturated Fat: 5g; Total Carbs: 11g; Fiber: 2g; Net Carbs: 3g; Protein: 10g; Sodium: 334mg; Sweetener: 6g

Macros: Fat: 73%; Carbs: 8%; Protein: 19%

Blueberry-Orange Scones

Dairy-Free, Extra Low-Carb, Gluten-Free, Low-Sodium, Vegetarian

MAKES 4 SCONES | PREP TIME: 10 MINUTES | COOK TIME: 25 MINUTES

If you are looking for a decadent breakfast treat, this is the recipe for you! This basic scone recipe allows for so many variations. Make this recipe "chocolate banana" by swapping the orange extract for banana extract and the blueberries for sugar-free chocolate chips. The possibilities are endless.

1½ cups almond flour

3 tablespoons granulated sugar substitute

Grated zest of 1 orange

¼ teaspoon baking powder

¼ teaspoon sea salt

1 large egg, at room temperature

2 tablespoons coconut oil, melted

¼ teaspoon orange extract

¼ cup blueberries

1 teaspoon powdered sugar substitute

1. Preheat the oven to 350°F. Line a baking sheet with parchment paper.

2. In a medium bowl, mix together the almond flour, sugar substitute, orange zest, baking powder, and salt until well combined.

3. Add the egg, oil, and orange extract. Mix until well incorporated. Gently fold in the blueberries.

4. Place the dough on the prepared baking sheet and form into a ½-inch-thick round. Cut the round into quarters and pull them about 1 inch apart on the baking sheet.

5. Bake for 20 to 25 minutes, until golden brown. Allow to cool on the baking sheet.

6. When serving, sprinkle each scone with a bit of powdered sugar substitute.

COOKING TIP: When all the ingredients are mixed together properly, the mixture should have the consistency of a cookie dough. When forming into a round, wetting your hands helps keep the dough from sticking.

Per serving (1 scone): Calories: 288; Total fat: 26g; Saturated Fat: 8g; Total Carbs: 18g; Fiber: 5g; Net Carbs: 4g; Protein: 9g; Sodium: 135mg; Sweetener: 9g

Macros: Fat: 75%; Carbs: 13%; Protein: 12%

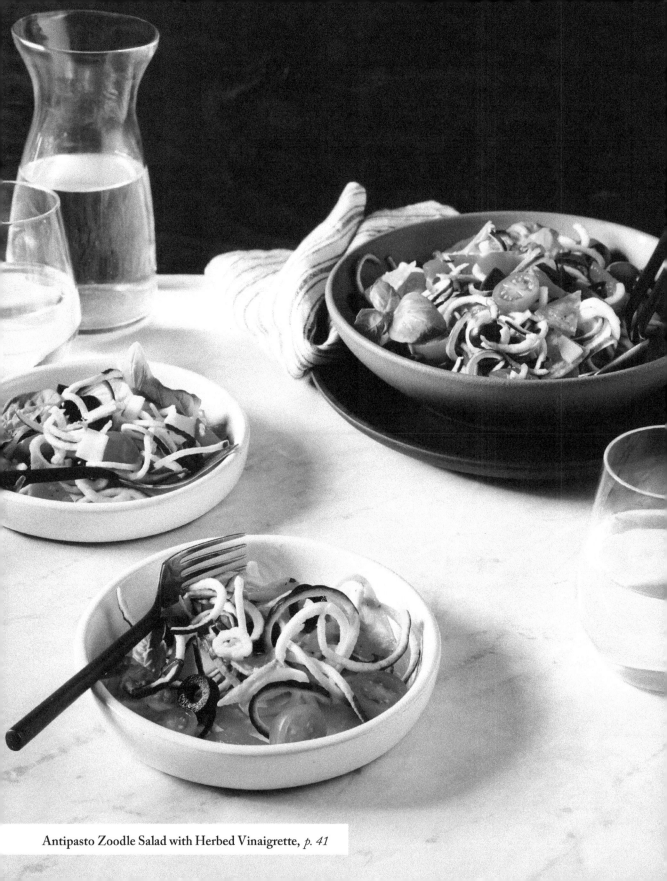

Antipasto Zoodle Salad with Herbed Vinaigrette, *p. 41*

Chapter Three

SOUPS, SALADS, AND SANDWICHES

Chipotle Vegetable and Bean Soup

Dairy-Free, Gluten-Free, Low-Sodium, Vegan

SERVES 2 | PREP TIME: 15 MINUTES | COOK TIME: 25 MINUTES

Edamame is an incredible replacement for high-carb beans and lentils. A young green soybean found in many East Asian cuisines, edamame have become increasingly popular in the United States and can be found shelled in the freezer section of most supermarkets. The smokiness from the chipotle powder gives this soup a rich, earthy flavor you are sure to love.

2 tablespoons extra-virgin olive oil
1 celery stalk, thinly sliced
1 small carrot, chopped
½ white onion, chopped
3 garlic cloves, thinly sliced
2 cups vegetable stock
1 (14.5-ounce) can diced tomatoes, undrained

1 cup chopped kale
½ cup frozen shelled edamame, thawed
½ cup bite-size pieces green beans
½ tablespoon chipotle powder
Sea salt

Freshly ground black pepper
1 tablespoon roughly chopped fresh cilantro
1 lime, halved

1. In a small soup pot, warm the oil over medium-low heat. Add the celery, carrot, and onion and cook for 7 to 9 minutes, stirring frequently, until the vegetables begin to brown. Add the garlic and cook for an additional 2 minutes, stirring occasionally, until tender.

2. Increase the heat to high and add the vegetable stock, tomatoes and their juices, kale, edamame, green beans, and chipotle powder and bring to a boil. Reduce the heat to low, cover, and simmer for 10 to 15 minutes, until the green beans are tender. Season with salt and pepper to taste.

3. To serve, divide the soup between two bowls and garnish with the cilantro and a squeeze of lime juice.

DIETARY SWAP: To lower the sodium levels even more, use low-sodium stock and no-salt-added diced tomatoes.

Per serving: Calories: 252; Total fat: 17g; Saturated Fat: 2g; Total Carbs: 23g; Fiber: 9g; Net Carbs: 14g; Protein: 8g; Sodium: 405mg; Sweetener: 0g

Macros: Fat: 57%; Carbs: 33%; Protein: 10%

Creamy Chicken and Spinach Soup

Extra Low-Carb, Gluten-Free, Low-Sodium

SERVES 2 | PREP TIME: 10 MINUTES | COOK TIME: 25 MINUTES

Creamy soups are the ultimate comfort meal, and this one will not disappoint! The fresh herbs brighten the soup and give it an Italian feel. Pair this soup with a small side salad and you're all set for a quick weeknight meal when you're pressed for time.

2 tablespoons extra-virgin olive oil

8 ounces boneless, skinless chicken thighs, cut into ½-inch pieces

1 celery stalk, thinly sliced

1 small carrot, chopped

½ white onion, chopped

3 garlic cloves, thinly sliced

2 cups low-sodium chicken stock

⅓ cup half-and-half

1 teaspoon chopped fresh thyme leaves

½ teaspoon chopped fresh rosemary

2 cups chopped fresh spinach

Sea salt

Freshly ground black pepper

2 tablespoons finely shaved Parmesan cheese, for serving

1. In a soup pot, heat the oil over medium-high heat. Add the chicken, celery, carrot, onion, and garlic and cook, stirring frequently, until the chicken begins to brown.

2. Increase the heat to high and add the chicken stock, half-and-half, thyme, and rosemary and bring to a boil. Reduce the heat to low, cover, and simmer for 10 to 15 minutes, until the chicken is fully cooked.

3. Stir in the spinach. Season with salt and pepper to taste.

4. Divide between two bowls, garnish with Parmesan, and serve.

DIETARY SWAP: Make this soup dairy-free by swapping the half-and-half with coconut cream and omitting the Parmesan.

Per serving: Calories: 480; Total fat: 39g; Saturated Fat: 11g; Total Carbs: 11g; Fiber: 2g; Net Carbs: 9g; Protein: 23g; Sodium: 326mg; Sweetener: 0g

Macros: Fat: 72%; Carbs: 8%; Protein: 20%

Shrimp and Andouille Sausage Gumbo

Dairy-Free, Extra Low-Carb, Gluten-Free

SERVES 2 | PREP TIME: 10 MINUTES | COOK TIME: 25 MINUTES

Gumbo can be considered the signature soup of Louisiana. It's often slow cooked and served on a bed of rice on Sundays down in the bayou. Serve this gumbo over a bed of riced cauliflower to mimic the traditional version. If you don't like shrimp, feel free to swap in chicken, but add it in step 1, along with the sausage.

½ tablespoon extra-virgin olive oil

8 ounces andouille sausage, cut into ½-inch-thick slices

½ yellow onion, chopped

½ green bell pepper, chopped

2 celery stalks, chopped

2 garlic cloves, minced

1 (14.5-ounce) can diced tomatoes, undrained

1 cup beef stock

1 tablespoon Cajun seasoning

1 teaspoon filé powder (optional)

⅛ teaspoon cayenne pepper (optional)

8 ounces large shrimp, peeled and deveined

Sea salt

Freshly ground black pepper

1. In a soup pot, heat the oil over medium-high heat. Add the sausage, onion, bell pepper, celery, and garlic and cook for 7 to 9 minutes, stirring frequently, until the sausage begins to brown.

2. Increase the heat to high and add the diced tomatoes and their juices, beef stock, Cajun seasoning, filé powder (if using), and cayenne (if using) and bring to a boil.

3. Reduce the heat to low, add the shrimp, cover, and simmer for 10 to 15 minutes, until the shrimp is fully cooked. Season with salt and black pepper to taste.

4. Divide between two bowls and serve hot.

COOKING TIP: Make your own Cajun seasoning using ¼ teaspoon smoked paprika, ¼ teaspoon dried thyme, ½ teaspoon onion powder, ½ teaspoon garlic powder, ½ teaspoon dried oregano, and ¼ teaspoon ground black pepper.

Per serving: Calories: 546; Total fat: 37g; Saturated Fat: 12g; Total Carbs: 15g; Fiber: 5g; Net Carbs: 10g; Protein: 39g; Sodium: 1,521mg; Sweetener: 0g

Macros: Fat: 61%; Carbs: 11%; Protein: 28%

Ginger Sesame Pork Soup

Dairy-Free, Extra Low-Carb

SERVES 2 | PREP TIME: 10 MINUTES | COOK TIME: 15 MINUTES

This healthy, easy-to-prepare, broth-based soup will quickly become a weeknight favorite you can have on the table in less than 30 minutes. Ginger offers many wonderful health benefits for the body, including anti-inflammatory properties, so don't hesitate to garnish your soup with some extra fresh ginger before eating. Use the leftover bok choy stems for a quick stir-fry dinner or add them to your favorite soup.

½ tablespoon avocado oil or extra-virgin olive oil
1 teaspoon sesame oil
8 ounces ground pork
2 small carrots, diced
1½ teaspoons minced peeled fresh ginger

4 cups chicken stock
2 tablespoons soy sauce
1 cup halved sugar snap peas
1 cup thinly sliced bok choy leaves
Sea salt

Freshly ground black pepper
½ jalapeño, seeded and thinly sliced
½ cup chopped fresh cilantro
Juice of 1 lime

1. In a soup pot, heat both oils over medium-high heat. Add the pork, carrots, and ginger and cook for 5 to 7 minutes, stirring frequently, until the pork begins to brown.

2. Increase the heat to high, add the chicken stock and soy sauce, and bring to a boil. Reduce the heat to low, add the sugar snap peas, cover, and simmer for 10 minutes, or until the peas are tender.

3. Stir in the bok choy leaves and season with salt and pepper to taste.

4. Divide between two bowls and serve each garnished with jalapeño, cilantro, and lime juice.

DIETARY SWAP: Replace the ground pork with firm cubed tofu and the chicken stock with vegetable stock for a vegan version.

Per serving: Calories: 414; Total fat: 30g; Saturated Fat: 10g; Total Carbs: 14g; Fiber: 4g; Net Carbs: 10g; Protein: 23g; Sodium: 1,070mg; Sweetener: 0g

Macros: Fat: 65%; Carbs: 12%; Protein: 23%

Strawberry, Mint, and Avocado Salad

Extra Low-Carb, Gluten-Free, Low-Sodium, Vegetarian

SERVES 2 | PREP TIME: 10 MINUTES

Sweet strawberries and fresh mint always pair well together, but adding the avocado completely transforms this salad into something quite spectacular. This salad is so healthy, fresh, and flavorful, and it can easily be made into a heartier meal by topping with grilled fish, tofu, or chicken.

¼ cup avocado oil

2 tablespoons fresh lime juice

Sea salt

Freshly ground black pepper

6 cups baby spinach

½ cup sliced strawberries

1 avocado, diced

2 ounces goat cheese, crumbled

¼ cup thinly sliced fresh mint

¼ cup slivered almonds, toasted

1. In a small bowl, whisk together the oil and lime juice and season with salt and pepper to taste. Set aside.

2. Divide the spinach between two plates. Dividing evenly, top with the strawberries, avocado, goat cheese, mint, and almonds.

3. Drizzle the dressing over the salads right before serving.

COOKING TIP: To create a creamier dressing, instead of whisking together the ingredients by hand, pulse all the ingredients together in a blender or whisk with a hand mixer.

Per serving: Calories: 619; Total fat: 56g; Saturated Fat: 11g; Total Carbs: 23g; Fiber: 14g; Net Carbs: 9g; Protein: 15g; Sodium: 286mg; Sweetener: 0g

Macros: Fat: 78%; Carbs: 14%; Protein: 8%

Peach and Tomato Caprese Salad

Gluten-Free, Low-Sodium, Vegetarian

SERVES 2 | PREP TIME: 10 MINUTES

The sweetness from the ripe juicy peaches and balsamic vinegar will make you think you are eating dessert instead of a salad. You can turn this dish into a great appetizer by leaving out the mixed greens, slicing the tomatoes, peach, and mozzarella instead of cubing them, and plating on a nice platter—it's sure to wow your dinner guests!

¼ cup extra-virgin olive oil

2 tablespoons balsamic vinegar

Sea salt

Freshly ground black pepper

6 cups mixed greens

2 large heirloom tomatoes, cut into ½-inch pieces

1 peach, halved, pitted, cut into ½-inch pieces

4 ounces fresh mozzarella cheese, cut into ½-inch pieces

¼ cup thinly sliced fresh basil

1. In a small bowl, whisk together the oil and vinegar. Season with salt and pepper to taste. Set aside.

2. Divide the mixed greens between two plates. Dividing evenly, top with the heirloom tomatoes, peaches, mozzarella, and basil.

3. Drizzle the dressing over the salads right before serving.

COOKING TIP: If the tomatoes are not quite as sweet and ripe as you'd like, toss them lightly in salt and allow to rest in the refrigerator for about 30 minutes prior to assembling the salad. This will help bring out the natural juices and enhance their sweetness.

Per serving: Calories: 507; Total fat: 41g; Saturated Fat: 11g; Total Carbs: 22g; Fiber: 5g; Net Carbs: 17g; Protein: 17g; Sodium: 455mg; Sweetener: 0g

Macros: Fat: 71%; Carbs: 16%; Protein: 13%

Cucumber and Red Onion Summer Salad

Extra Low-Carb, Gluten-Free, Low-Sodium, Vegetarian
SERVES 2 | PREP TIME: 15 MINUTES, PLUS 30 MINUTES TO CHILL

This fresh, tangy, and creamy cucumber salad is my ma's recipe—she always prepared it when we grilled out. It pairs well with grilled steaks, burgers, grilled chicken—all your cookout favorites! Triple or quadruple the recipe and bring this to your next potluck barbecue, and you'll be welcomed back with open arms. I do find that the longer the cucumber marinates in the dressing, the better it tastes, so if you have the time to let it chill for more than 30 minutes, do it.

- ½ cup sour cream
- 1 tablespoon chopped fresh dill
- 1 teaspoon apple cider vinegar
- ½ teaspoon granulated sugar substitute
- ½ teaspoon freshly ground black pepper
- ¼ teaspoon sea salt
- 1 English cucumber, thinly sliced
- ¼ red onion, thinly sliced

In a medium bowl, mix the sour cream, dill, vinegar, sugar substitute, pepper, and salt. Add the cucumber and red onion and mix well. Refrigerate for at least 30 minutes prior to serving.

DIETARY SWAP: Swap out the sour cream for unsweetened coconut yogurt to make this dish vegan and dairy-free.

Per serving: Calories: 138; Total fat: 11g; Saturated Fat: 7g; Total Carbs: 8g; Fiber: 1g; Net Carbs: 7g; Protein: 2g; Sodium: 263mg; Sweetener: 1g

Macros: Fat: 73%; Carbs: 21%; Protein: 6%

Antipasto Zoodle Salad with Herbed Vinaigrette

Extra Low-Carb, Gluten-Free

SERVES 2 | PREP TIME: 20 MINUTES

This cold antipasto salad is perfect for a hot summer meal when you just can't bear the thought of cooking. Ditch the cold pasta for "zoodles," zucchini that has been spiralized to mimic spaghetti. Not only does this make the dish healthier, it's also more colorful and fun to eat!

¼ cup extra-virgin olive oil

2 tablespoons red wine vinegar

2 teaspoons minced garlic

1 teaspoon chopped fresh oregano

1 teaspoon chopped fresh basil, plus more for garnish

Sea salt

Freshly ground black pepper

2 medium zucchini, spiralized

8 slices hard salami, roughly chopped

4 slices provolone cheese, roughly chopped

½ cup halved grape tomatoes

¼ cup sliced roasted red peppers

¼ cup pitted black olives, sliced

1. In a small bowl, whisk together the oil, vinegar, garlic, oregano, and basil. Season with salt and black pepper to taste.

2. In a large bowl, combine the zucchini, salami, provolone, tomatoes, roasted red peppers, and olives. Mix the dressing into the vegetables and refrigerate for 10 minutes.

3. Divide between two plates and garnish with fresh basil.

COOKING TIP: If you do not have a spiralizer, you can make zoodles with a vegetable peeler. Start from the top of the zucchini and peel all the way down to the bottom. You'll get zucchini ribbons that work just as well.

Per serving: Calories: 653; Total fat: 57g; Saturated Fat: 18g; Total Carbs: 12g; Fiber: 3g; Net Carbs: 9g; Protein: 26g; Sodium: 1,300mg; Sweetener: 0g

Macros: Fat: 77%; Carbs: 7%; Protein: 16%

Peppercorn Ranch Kale Salad with Toasted Walnuts

Extra Low-Carb, Gluten-Free, Low-Sodium

SERVES 2 | PREP TIME: 30 MINUTES

Replacing the traditional romaine in this salad with kale adds so many more nutrients. Kale is much higher in vitamin C, vitamin K, potassium, and calcium—your body will definitely thank you.

½ cup walnut halves

4 to 6 cups kale, stems removed and cut into bite-size pieces

Juice of 1 lemon

Sea salt

¼ cup Sugar-Free Ranch Dressing (page 145)

½ teaspoon coarsely cracked black pepper

2 tablespoons shaved Parmesan cheese

1. In a dry skillet, toast the walnuts over medium heat, stirring frequently, for about 5 minutes. Remove from the skillet and set aside.

2. In a large bowl, gently massage the kale with the lemon juice and a pinch of salt for 2 minutes. This will help soften the kale.

3. In a small bowl, mix together the ranch dressing and pepper until well combined. Add the dressing to the kale and toss well until the kale is evenly coated.

4. Divide between two bowls. Top with the Parmesan and toasted walnuts.

COOKING TIP: To remove the stems and midribs from the kale, hold a leaf up by the stem with one hand and with the other hand strip the leaf off the stem, gently moving your hand downward until the two leaf halves fall off.

Per serving: Calories: 333; Total fat: 29g; Saturated Fat: 5g; Total Carbs: 10g; Fiber: 3g; Net Carbs: 7g; Protein: 8g; Sodium: 297mg; Sweetener: 0g

Macros: Fat: 78%; Carbs: 12%; Protein: 10%

Shrimp with Cilantro Ranch Slaw Lettuce Wraps

Gluten-Free

SERVES 2 | PREP TIME: 25 MINUTES | COOK TIME: 5 MINUTES

This simple recipe just explodes with a contrast of amazing flavors, textures, and nutrients. Shrimp is a great protein that is low in calories and rich in vitamins and omega-3 fatty acids.

1 pound medium shrimp, peeled and deveined
2 garlic cloves, minced
2 teaspoons ground cumin
2 teaspoons chili powder
1½ teaspoons sea salt, divided

1 teaspoon freshly ground black pepper, divided
½ head cabbage, shredded
1 small carrot, shredded
2½ tablespoons chopped fresh cilantro, divided
1 lime, halved, divided

¼ cup Sugar-Free Ranch Dressing (page 145)
1 tablespoon avocado oil
4 romaine lettuce leaves
1 avocado, chopped

1. In a bowl, combine the shrimp, garlic, cumin, chili powder, 1 teaspoon of salt, and ½ teaspoon of pepper and mix well to evenly coat the shrimp. Set aside.

2. In a separate bowl, combine the cabbage, carrot, 1 tablespoon of cilantro, juice of ½ lime, and the ranch dressing. Mix well and season with the remaining ½ teaspoon of salt and ½ teaspoon of pepper.

3. In a large skillet, heat the oil over medium-high heat. Add the shrimp and cook for 2 to 3 minutes per side, until pink, firm, and cooked throughout. Squeeze the juice from the remaining ½ lime over the shrimp.

4. Set 2 lettuce leaves each on two plates. Evenly divide the coleslaw among the lettuce leaves. Top each lettuce leaf with one-quarter of the shrimp and avocado.

COOKING TIP: When mincing garlic, sprinkle with about ⅛ teaspoon sea salt. This will help keep the garlic in place and create a more even mince.

Per serving: Calories: 664; Total fat: 36g; Saturated Fat: 7g; Total Carbs: 31g; Fiber: 16g; Net Carbs: 15g; Protein: 54g; Sodium: 1,247mg; Sweetener: 0g

Macros: Fat: 48%; Carbs: 19%; Protein: 33%

Curry and Grape Chicken Salad Lettuce Cups

Extra Low-Carb, Gluten-Free, Low-Sodium

SERVES 2 | PREP TIME: 15 MINUTES | COOK TIME: 15 MINUTES

This childhood favorite was often served at our kitchen table. The earthy flavor of the curry and the sweet grapes play so well together. Then the crunch from the almonds brings it all together to make your taste buds dance. This tasty salad will soon become a staple at your kitchen table, too.

1 (6- to 8-ounce) boneless, skinless chicken breast, cut into ¼-inch cubes

¼ cup mayonnaise

2 tablespoons sour cream

2 tablespoons halved red grapes

1 tablespoon sliced almonds, toasted

1 teaspoon curry powder

¼ teaspoon sea salt

⅛ teaspoon ground white pepper

6 butter lettuce leaves

1. In a medium skillet or saucepan, combine the chicken and enough water to come halfway up the chicken. Bring to a low simmer over medium-high heat, cover, and cook the chicken for 10 to 15 minutes, until the juices run clear. Drain the poaching liquid and place the chicken in the refrigerator to cool for 15 to 20 minutes.

2. In a medium bowl, mix together the cooled chicken, mayonnaise, sour cream, grapes, almonds, curry powder, salt, and white pepper until well incorporated.

3. Set 3 lettuce leaves each on two plates. Evenly divide the chicken salad among the lettuce leaves, taco style, and serve.

COOKING TIP: Save on cooking time by using a rotisserie chicken from your local supermarket.

Per serving: Calories: 376; Total fat: 31g; Saturated Fat: 7g; Total Carbs: 4g; Fiber: 1g; Net Carbs: 3g; Protein: 19g; Sodium: 469mg; Sweetener: 0g

Macros: Fat: 75%; Carbs: 4%; Protein: 21%

Open-Faced Mediterranean Chicken Salad Sandwiches

Extra Low-Carb, Gluten-Free, Low-Sodium

SERVES 2 | PREP TIME: 20 MINUTES | COOK TIME: 15 MINUTES

When I would visit my grandmother as a teen, she would always make this chicken salad and serve it on a croissant or a buttery roll because she knew it was my favorite. Using a homemade low-carb bread makes this chicken salad sandwich a go-to meal for me.

1 (6- to 8-ounce) boneless, skinless chicken breast, cut into ¼-inch cubes

4 pitted green olives, sliced

1 tablespoon minced red onion

2 tablespoons extra-virgin olive oil

1 tablespoon red wine vinegar

1 tablespoon finely sliced fresh basil

1 tablespoon chopped fresh oregano

1 tablespoon grated Parmesan cheese

1 garlic clove, minced

Sea salt

Freshly ground black pepper

2 "slices" Soft and Fluffy Sandwich Bread (page 136)

½ cup mixed greens

1. In a medium skillet or saucepan, combine the chicken and enough water to come halfway up the sides of the chicken. Bring to a low simmer over medium-high heat, cover, and cook for 10 to 15 minutes, until the juices run clear. Drain off the poaching liquid and place in the refrigerator to cool for 15 to 20 minutes.

2. In a medium bowl, combine the chicken, olives, onion, oil, vinegar, basil, oregano, Parmesan, and garlic. Mix until well incorporated. Season with salt and pepper to taste.

3. Place 1 slice of bread each on two plates. Top with the mixed greens. Dividing evenly, top the greens with the chicken salad.

COOKING TIP: Poaching chicken is the easiest way to ensure the meat is really moist, which is ideal for these types of salads.

Per serving: Calories: 440; Total fat: 35g; Saturated Fat: 7g; Total Carbs: 4g; Fiber: 2g; Net Carbs: 2g; Protein: 24g; Sodium: 391mg; Sweetener: 0g

Macros: Fat: 72%; Carbs: 6%; Protein: 22%

French Onion and Spinach Grilled Cheese Sandwiches

Extra Low-Carb, Gluten-Free, Vegetarian

SERVES 2 | PREP TIME: 15 MINUTES | COOK TIME: 40 MINUTES

French onion soup was a staple in my St. Louis childhood home. If we were not preparing it ourselves, we were eating it at a popular local restaurant. Transforming this flavorful soup into a sandwich offers the opportunity to experience the flavors more conveniently—although napkins are still necessary.

1 tablespoon extra-virgin olive oil

2 tablespoons butter, divided

1 large yellow onion, cut into ⅛-inch-thick slices

2 garlic cloves, chopped

Double recipe (4 "slices") Soft and Fluffy Sandwich Bread (page 136)

1 tablespoon mayonnaise

1 cup shredded Gruyère or Swiss cheese

2 cups chopped baby spinach

1. In a large skillet, heat the oil and 1 tablespoon of butter over medium-low heat. Add the onion and garlic and cook for 25 to 30 minutes, stirring occasionally to prevent burning.

2. Meanwhile, use the remaining 1 tablespoon of butter to spread on one side of each slice of bread.

3. In another skillet, place 2 slices of bread, butter-side down. Top each slice with ½ tablespoon of mayonnaise, ¼ cup of Gruyère, half the caramelized onions, and ½ cup of spinach. Top each with another ¼ cup of cheese and close the sandwiches with the remaining slices of bread, butter-side up.

4. Cover, set the pan over medium-high heat, and cook for 1 to 2 minutes per side, or until golden brown and the cheese is melted.

5. Cut in half and serve hot.

COOKING TIP: When caramelizing onions, it is important to use a butter-and-oil combination to prevent the butter from burning. Caramelize the onions at a slow and steady pace to produce a deep and rich flavor.

Per serving: Calories: 749; Total fat: 65g; Saturated Fat: 23g; Total Carbs: 13g; Fiber: 4g; Net Carbs: 9g; Protein: 28g; Sodium: 908mg; Sweetener: 0g

Macros: Fat: 78%; Carbs: 7%; Protein: 15%

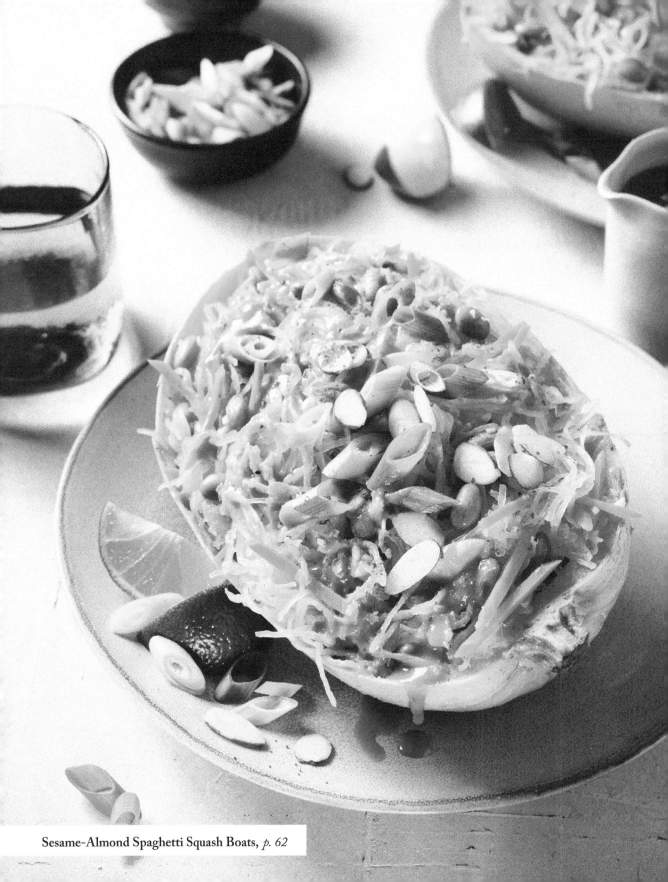

Sesame-Almond Spaghetti Squash Boats, *p. 62*

Chapter Four

MEATLESS MAINS

Smoky Edamame and Sweet Potato Chili

Dairy-Free, Gluten-Free, Low-Sodium, Vegan

SERVES 2 | PREP TIME: 10 MINUTES | COOK TIME: 25 MINUTES

The contrast between the sweet potatoes and the rich, earthy chocolate in this delightful chili will knock your socks off. Edamame is a fabulous low-carb alternative to your standard chili bean, and it's also packed with a substantial amount of protein to keep your hunger at bay.

1 tablespoon avocado oil or extra-virgin olive oil

¼ sweet potato, cut into ¼-inch chunks

¼ white onion, chopped

1 poblano pepper, seeded and diced

2 garlic cloves, minced

2 cups unsalted vegetable stock

1 (14.5-ounce) can crushed tomatoes

½ cup frozen shelled edamame, thawed

1 ounce unsweetened baker's chocolate, roughly chopped

1 tablespoon ground cumin

1 tablespoon chili powder

1 teaspoon chipotle powder

Sea salt

Freshly ground black pepper

1. In a medium saucepan, heat the oil over medium-high heat. Add the sweet potato, onion, poblano, and garlic and cook for 5 to 7 minutes, until the onion and sweet potato begin to caramelize.

2. Reduce the heat to medium and add the vegetable stock, crushed tomatoes, edamame, chocolate, cumin, chili powder, and chipotle powder. Simmer for 10 to 15 minutes, until the sweet potatoes are tender.

3. Season with salt and pepper to taste. Divide between two bowls and serve.

COOKING TIP: This chili can also be prepared in a small slow cooker. Add all the ingredients, set on low for 4 hours, and walk away.

Per serving: Calories: 327; Total fat: 18g; Saturated Fat: 6g; Total Carbs: 37g; Fiber: 11g; Net Carbs: 26g; Protein: 11g; Sodium: 306mg; Sweetener: 0g

Macros: Fat: 48%; Carbs: 41%; Protein: 11%

Chipotle, Poblano, and Tomato Casserole

Gluten-Free, Low-Sodium, Vegetarian

SERVES 2 | PREP TIME: 10 MINUTES | COOK TIME: 25 MINUTES

This casserole reminds me of taco pie, but without the carbs. The smoky flavors from the poblano and chipotle are what make this dish stand out. This is a great choice for your next Taco Tuesday. Use the leftover canned chipotle peppers to make a batch of home-made salsa by adding onion, tomato, and chopped fresh cilantro.

Nonstick cooking spray

1 tablespoon avocado oil or extra-virgin olive oil

2 cups riced cauliflower

½ red bell pepper, diced

¼ white onion, diced

½ poblano pepper, seeded and diced

1 teaspoon adobo sauce from canned chipotle peppers

½ teaspoon ground cumin

½ teaspoon chili powder

8 cherry tomatoes, halved

½ cup shredded sharp Cheddar cheese, divided

1 tablespoon chopped fresh cilantro

1 avocado, sliced

1. Preheat the oven to 350°F. Mist a mini loaf pan with cooking spray.

2. In large skillet, heat the oil over medium-high heat. Add the cauliflower, bell pepper, onion, and poblano and cook for 2 to 3 minutes, until the onion starts to soften.

3. Add the adobo sauce, cumin, and chili powder and cook for an additional minute. Remove from the heat and allow to cool for 5 minutes. Stir in the cherry tomatoes and ¼ cup of Cheddar.

4. Evenly spread the mixture into the prepared loaf pan. Top with the remaining ¼ cup of Cheddar. Bake for 10 to 15 minutes, until the cheese is slightly browned.

5. Scoop the mixture onto two plates and garnish with the cilantro. Serve the avocado slices on the side.

COOKING TIP: Don't skip sautéing the vegetables before baking them. This step caramelizes the veggies and enhances their flavors.

Per serving: Calories: 423; Total fat: 33g; Saturated Fat: 9g; Total Carbs: 25g; Fiber: 13g; Net Carbs: 12g; Protein: 14g; Sodium: 257mg; Sweetener: 0g

Macros: Fat: 67%; Carbs: 21%; Protein: 12%

Mozzarella Portobello Mushroom Stacks

Gluten-Free, Vegetarian

SERVES 2 | PREP TIME: 10 MINUTES | COOK TIME: 30 MINUTES

This dish totally screams summer to me! The fresh mozzarella, fresh basil, and juicy tomatoes are a combination that just can't be beat. If you can't get fresh mozzarella, shredded works just as well.

1 tablespoon avocado oil or extra-virgin olive oil
½ white onion, minced
3 garlic cloves, chopped
1 (14.5-ounce) can diced tomatoes, drained
2 tablespoons finely chopped fresh oregano

Sea salt
Freshly ground black pepper
2 large portobello mushrooms, stems and gills removed
1 small zucchini, thinly sliced

1 tomato, thinly sliced
4 ounces fresh mozzarella cheese, sliced
6 large fresh basil leaves, thinly sliced, plus more for garnish

1. Preheat the oven to 350°F.

2. In an ovenproof medium skillet, heat the oil over medium-high heat for 30 seconds. Add the onion and garlic and cook for 2 minutes, or until the onion begins to brown. Add the tomatoes and oregano and cook for an additional minute. Season with salt and pepper to taste.

3. Place the mushrooms, stemmed-side up, in the skillet. Season each with a pinch of salt and pepper. Place a spoonful of sauce into the cavity of each mushroom. Top each mushroom with one-quarter of the zucchini slices, tomato slices, and mozzarella slices. Place 3 basil leaves on each mushroom. Repeat the zucchini and tomato layers, and top each mushroom stack with the remaining mozzarella.

4. Bake for 20 to 25 minutes, until the cheese is melted and the mushrooms are al dente.

5. Serve, garnished with basil.

Per serving: Calories: 329; Total fat: 21g; Saturated Fat: 9g; Total Carbs: 21g; Fiber: 7g; Net Carbs: 14g; Protein: 18g; Sodium: 690mg; Sweetener: 0g

Macros: Fat: 56%; Carbs: 23%; Protein: 21%

Edamame Falafel with Lemony Garlic Aioli

Dairy-Free, Gluten-Free, Vegetarian

SERVES 2 | PREP TIME: 15 MINUTES | COOK TIME: 35 MINUTES

This meatless option can be served in so many ways. These flavorful protein-packed patties work well as an appetizer, as a salad topper, or swaddled in a lettuce leaf.

Nonstick cooking spray

1 tablespoon extra-virgin olive oil

½ cup chopped white onions

3 garlic cloves, 2 chopped and 1 minced

3 ounces white mushrooms, roughly chopped

1 small carrot, chopped

½ cup frozen shelled edamame, thawed

¼ cup almond flour

2 tablespoons walnuts

2 tablespoons chopped fresh parsley

½ teaspoon smoked paprika

½ teaspoon ground cumin

½ teaspoon sea salt

½ teaspoon freshly ground black pepper

¼ cup mayonnaise

Juice of ½ lemon

1. Preheat the oven to 400°F. Mist a large baking sheet with cooking spray.

2. In a skillet, heat the oil over medium heat. Add the onions and chopped garlic and cook for 3 to 5 minutes, until the onions begin to caramelize.

3. Transfer the mixture to a food processor and add the mushrooms, carrot, edamame, almond flour, walnuts, parsley, paprika, cumin, salt, and pepper. Pulse until the mixture has the texture of small grains.

4. Form the mixture into 6 patties each 2½ inches in diameter and place on the prepared baking sheet. Bake for 30 to 35 minutes, until they feel spongy.

5. In a small bowl, mix together the mayonnaise, lemon juice, and minced garlic until well combined.

6. Serve 3 patties per person with the aioli on the side for dipping.

COOKING TIP: Make sure not to overprocess the falafel mixture or you'll have hummus instead.

Per serving: Calories: 450; Total fat: 40g; Saturated Fat: 5g; Total Carbs: 17g; Fiber: 6g; Net Carbs: 11g; Protein: 10g; Sodium: 667mg; Sweetener: 0g

Macros: Fat: 78%; Carbs: 14%; Protein: 8%

Vegetable Pesto Pizza

Gluten-Free, Vegetarian

SERVES 2 | PREP TIME: 10 MINUTES | COOK TIME: 35 MINUTES

This pizza is loaded with vibrant pesto, fresh tomatoes, and creamy ricotta, and I bet it will have you passing on traditional pizza from here on out. Why grab a jar of pizza sauce when you can use fresh quality ingredients from your garden or the produce section?

"Fathead" Pizza Crust (page 137)

1 tablespoon extra-virgin olive oil, plus 2 teaspoons

½ cup sliced mushrooms

¼ white onion, thinly sliced

2 garlic cloves, minced

¼ cup pesto

10 ounces frozen chopped spinach, thawed and excess water squeezed out

½ cup quartered cherry tomatoes

⅓ cup ricotta cheese

2 cups baby arugula

1. Preheat the oven to 425°F. Line a baking sheet with parchment paper.

2. Assemble and bake the pizza crust as directed. Leave the oven on.

3. Meanwhile, in a medium skillet, heat 1 tablespoon of oil over medium-high heat. Add the mushrooms, onion, and garlic and cook for 5 to 7 minutes, until the onion becomes tender.

4. Spread the pesto evenly over the baked pizza crust. Top with the onion and mushroom mixture, chopped spinach, and cherry tomatoes. Dollop the ricotta across the top.

5. Bake for 8 to 10 minutes, until the tomatoes and cheese begin to brown.

6. Scatter the arugula over the pizza and drizzle with the remaining 2 teaspoons of olive oil. Slice into quarters and serve hot.

COOKING TIP: Don't skip quartering the cherry tomatoes! The smaller they are cut, the deeper they will caramelize, which adds natural sweetness to the pizza.

Per serving: Calories: 968; Total fat: 77g; Saturated Fat: 24g; Total Carbs: 24g; Fiber: 10g; Net Carbs: 14g; Protein: 45g; Sodium: 1,338mg; Sweetener: 0g

Macros: Fat: 72%; Carbs: 9%; Protein: 19%

Loaded Barbecue Roasted Cabbage Steaks

Gluten-Free, Vegetarian

SERVES 2 | PREP TIME: 10 MINUTES | COOK TIME: 35 MINUTES

When I lived in Texas, I would frequent the barbecue restaurants and order a loaded baked potato. So, this is my version of a Texas-style barbecue potato. Replacing the potato with the cabbage greatly decreases the carbs and calories. This recipe would also work well with mashed cauliflower and served as a side dish.

½ head cabbage, sliced into 4 (1-inch-thick) steaks

2 tablespoons avocado oil

1 teaspoon freshly ground black pepper

½ teaspoon sea salt

2 tablespoons sugar-free barbecue sauce

½ cup shredded sharp Cheddar cheese

1 avocado, diced

½ jalapeño, seeded and thinly sliced

1 scallion, chopped

2 tablespoons sour cream

½ cup chopped fresh cilantro

1. Preheat the oven to 400°F. Line a baking sheet with parchment paper.

2. Drizzle both sides of the cabbage steaks with the oil and season with the pepper and salt. Bake for 15 minutes, then flip and bake for an additional 15 minutes. The cabbage should be browned with a tender center.

3. Remove the cabbage steaks and turn the oven to broil.

4. Dividing evenly, top each cabbage steak with the barbecue sauce and Cheddar. Broil for 3 to 5 minutes, until the cheese is melted.

5. Plate 2 steaks per serving and top with the avocado, jalapeño, scallion, sour cream, and cilantro.

COOKING TIP: Make your own sugar-free barbecue sauce using my Sugar-Free Ketchup recipe (page 143), following the barbecue sauce variation.

Per serving: Calories: 493; Total fat: 41g; Saturated Fat: 12g; Total Carbs: 24g; Fiber: 13g; Net Carbs: 11g; Protein: 13g; Sodium: 691mg; Sweetener: 0g

Macros: Fat: 73%; Carbs: 17%; Protein: 10%

Balsamic Rosemary Roasted Squash and Root Vegetables

Dairy-Free, Gluten-Free, Vegan

SERVES 2 | PREP TIME: 15 MINUTES | COOK TIME: 50 MINUTES

I like to pair balsamic vinegar with root vegetables because of the contrast of the sweet and earthy flavors. This recipe is quite versatile, so don't hesitate to mix up your vegetables and use what's in season.

1 small acorn squash, halved, seeded, peeled, and cut into ½-inch pieces

1 small beet, peeled and cut into ½-inch pieces

1 small carrot, peeled and cut into ½-inch pieces

4 ounces radishes, quartered

½ red onion, cut into ½-inch wedges

¼ cup extra-virgin olive oil

8 garlic cloves, peeled

2 tablespoons balsamic vinegar

1 teaspoon sea salt

1 teaspoon freshly ground black pepper

1 tablespoon chopped fresh rosemary

1. Preheat the oven to 400°F. Line a baking sheet with parchment paper.

2. In a large bowl, toss together the acorn squash, beet, carrot, radishes, onion, oil, garlic cloves, vinegar, salt, and pepper until the vegetables are evenly coated.

3. Spread the vegetables on the prepared baking sheet and roast for 35 minutes.

4. Sprinkle the rosemary on top and stir the veggies with a spatula. Bake for an additional 10 to 15 minutes, until tender.

5. Divide evenly between two plates and enjoy.

DIETARY SWAP: Make this dish lower in carbs by using more radishes and Brussels sprouts in place of the beet and carrot.

Per serving (2 cups): Calories: 400; Total fat: 27g; Saturated Fat: 4g; Total Carbs: 33g; Fiber: 8g; Net Carbs: 25g; Protein: 3g; Sodium: 1,165mg; Sweetener: 0g

Macros: Fat: 63%; Carbs: 34%; Protein: 3%

Fennel and Feta Shakshuka

Gluten-Free, Vegetarian

SERVES 2 | PREP TIME: 10 MINUTES | COOK TIME: 18 MINUTES

This is such a simple recipe that can be served at any meal. It's a statement dish that's fancy enough for entertaining, too. Use every part of the fennel by chopping up the fennel fronds and throwing them in a large salad to serve with this dish.

1 tablespoon extra-virgin olive oil

1 small bulb fennel, stalks and fronds removed, bulb thinly sliced

½ white onion, diced

½ red bell pepper, diced

½ jalapeño, seeded and chopped

1 (14.5-ounce) can diced fire-roasted tomatoes, undrained

¼ cup vegetable stock

1 teaspoon ground cumin

½ teaspoon smoked paprika

4 large eggs

½ cup crumbled feta cheese

Sea salt

Freshly ground black pepper

¼ cup chopped fresh parsley

1. In a large skillet, heat the oil over medium-high heat. Add the fennel and onion and cook for 3 minutes, stirring frequently, until they begin to soften. Add the bell pepper and jalapeño and cook for an additional 5 minutes, or until the fennel and onion begin to brown.

2. Add the tomatoes and their juices, vegetable stock, cumin, and smoked paprika and simmer for 5 minutes to reduce the sauce by about one-quarter.

3. Reduce the heat to low and gently crack the eggs atop the tomato sauce, evenly spread with the feta, and cover. Cook for 5 minutes, or until the egg whites are cooked and the yolks reach the desired doneness. Season with salt and black pepper to taste.

4. Dividing evenly, spoon into bowls and garnish with the parsley.

DIETARY SWAP: Make this dish vegan by replacing the feta with a few olives for brininess. It will be just as wonderful.

Per Serving: Calories: 400; Total fat: 25g; Saturated Fat: 10g; Total Carbs: 24g; Fiber: 9g; Net Carbs: 15g; Protein: 22g; Sodium: 870mg; Sweetener: 0g

Macros: Fat: 56%; Carbs: 22%; Protein: 22%

Herb and Lemon Roasted Vegetables

Dairy-Free, Gluten-Free, Vegan

SERVES 2 | PREP TIME: 10 MINUTES | COOK TIME: 35 MINUTES

This is such a simple and flavorful vegetable recipe that I'm sure it will be rotating on your menu quite often. Roasting the veggies enhances their sweetness and earthiness. Serve this with your favorite lean protein or throw the vegetables on top of a large green salad with my Raspberry Balsamic Vinaigrette (page 147).

8 Brussels sprouts, quartered

8 baby bella (cremini) mushrooms

1 medium carrot, cut into ¼-inch pieces

1 red bell pepper, cut into ½-inch-wide strips

1 head broccoli, cut into small florets

½ red onion, cut into ½-inch pieces

8 garlic cloves, peeled

2 tablespoons avocado oil or extra-virgin olive oil

1 teaspoon freshly ground black pepper

½ teaspoon sea salt

½ cup halved cherry tomatoes

1 tablespoon fresh thyme

2 teaspoons chopped fresh oregano

½ lemon

1. Preheat the oven to 400°F. Line a baking sheet with parchment paper.

2. On the prepared baking sheet, combine the Brussels sprouts, mushrooms, carrot, bell pepper, broccoli, onion, and garlic. Drizzle with the oil, season with the black pepper and salt, and gently toss to coat the vegetables. Roast for 15 to 20 minutes, until they begin to become tender.

3. Add the tomatoes, thyme, and oregano to the baking sheet, toss, and bake for an additional 15 minutes, or until the vegetables are browned.

4. Squeeze the lemon over the roasted veggies. Divide evenly and serve hot.

COOKING TIP: Cutting your veggies into roughly the same size will ensure that they roast evenly.

Per serving: Calories: 349; Total fat: 16g; Saturated Fat: 2g; Total Carbs: 45g; Fiber: 15g; Net Carbs: 30g; Protein: 15g; Sodium: 621mg; Sweetener: 0g

Macros: Fat: 48%; Carbs: 41%; Protein: 11%

Cauliflower and Kale Curry

Dairy-Free, Gluten-Free, Vegan

SERVES 2 | PREP TIME: 10 MINUTES | COOK TIME: 25 MINUTES

This vegan curry is rich in earthy, spicy flavors. Serve this over a bed of riced cauliflower or Shredded Cabbage Noodles (page 138) for a warm meal on a cold night.

1 tablespoon avocado oil or extra-virgin olive oil

½ white onion, diced

1 head cauliflower, cut into ½-inch pieces

2 garlic cloves, thinly sliced

1 tablespoon minced peeled fresh ginger

1 (14.5-ounce) can full-fat coconut milk

1 (14.5-ounce) can diced tomatoes, undrained

1 cup chopped kale

1 tablespoon curry powder

1 teaspoon ground cumin

½ teaspoon ground turmeric

½ teaspoon sea salt

½ teaspoon freshly ground pepper

Chopped fresh Thai basil or sweet basil

1 lime, halved

1. In a large skillet, heat the oil over medium-high heat. Add the onion and cook for 5 minutes, or until just tender. Add the cauliflower, garlic, and ginger and cook for 5 minutes, or until the cauliflower begins to slightly brown.

2. Reduce the heat to medium-low and add the coconut milk, diced tomatoes and their juices, kale, curry powder, cumin, turmeric, salt, and pepper. Cover and simmer for 15 to 20 minutes, until the cauliflower is fork-tender.

3. Serve garnished with basil, with a lime half for squeezing.

COOKING TIP: Sautéing the cauliflower prior to adding it to the liquid ingredients helps enhance its nutty, toasty flavors.

Per serving: Calories: 571; Total fat: 53g; Saturated Fat: 40g; Total Carbs: 27g; Fiber: 9g; Net Carbs: 18g; Protein: 10g; Sodium: 777mg; Sweetener: 0g

Macros: Fat: 78%; Carbs: 17%; Protein: 5%

Grilled Avocado and Vegetable Bowl with Tahini Sauce

Dairy-Free, Gluten-Free, Vegan

SERVES 2 | PREP TIME: 10 MINUTES | COOK TIME: 10 MINUTES

Avocados are a superfood loaded with potassium, fiber, and heart-healthy fats. You may think that because this is a vegetable bowl you'll be starving soon after eating, but the fat from the avocado and tahini is going to keep you full for hours.

Juice from 1 lemon

2 tablespoons water

1½ tablespoons tahini paste

1½ tablespoons avocado oil or extra-virgin olive oil, divided

2 garlic cloves, minced

1 avocado, halved and pitted

1 small zucchini, cut lengthwise into ¼-inch-thick slices

2 portobello mushrooms

1 small yellow squash, cut lengthwise into ¼-inch-thick slices

1 red bell pepper, cut vertically into 4 flat panels

1 teaspoon sea salt

1 teaspoon freshly ground black pepper

¼ cup chopped fresh cilantro

1. Preheat a grill.

2. In a small bowl, whisk the lemon juice, water, tahini paste, 1 tablespoon of oil, and the garlic. Set aside.

3. On a baking sheet or tray (something you can carry to the grill), season the avocado, zucchini, mushrooms, squash, and bell pepper with the salt and black pepper and drizzle with the remaining ½ tablespoon of oil.

4. Grill the avocado, cut-side down, for 4 to 6 minutes, until grill marks develop. Grill the vegetables for 2 to 4 minutes per side, until they develop grill marks and are al dente. Slice the mushrooms once they're cool enough to touch.

5. Dividing evenly, arrange the vegetables in two bowls. Scoop an avocado half onto each serving. Drizzle each bowl with 2½ tablespoons tahini dressing and garnish with the cilantro. (Save the remaining dressing for salad dressings; store in the refrigerator for up to 5 days.)

COOKING TIP: If you don't have a grill, broil on a baking sheet 6 to 7 inches from the broiler for 8 to 10 minutes, adding the avocado toward the end, until the veggies are golden brown and tender.

Per serving: Calories: 423; Total fat: 33g; Saturated Fat: 5g; Total Carbs: 30g; Fiber: 14g; Net Carbs: 16g; Protein: 10g; Sodium: 1,121mg; Sweetener: 0g

Macros: Fat: 67%; Carbs: 24%; Protein: 9%

Sesame-Almond Spaghetti Squash Boats

Dairy-Free, Vegan

SERVES 2 | PREP TIME: 10 MINUTES | COOK TIME: 50 MINUTES

Spaghetti squash is my go-to replacement for pasta and noodles. This dish is actually quite rich and creamy because of the tahini and sesame oil, so you won't miss the carbs at all.

1 small spaghetti squash, halved lengthwise and seeded

½ teaspoon sea salt, plus more to taste

½ teaspoon freshly ground black pepper, plus more to taste

2 tablespoons sesame oil, divided

2 tablespoons brown sugar substitute

1 lime, ½ juiced and ½ sliced into wedges

1 tablespoon reduced-sodium soy sauce

¼ cup tahini or nut butter

¼ teaspoon red pepper flakes

1 to 2 tablespoons hot water

½ cup frozen shelled edamame, thawed

¼ cup shredded carrots

½ tablespoon grated peeled fresh ginger

2 garlic cloves, chopped

¼ cup chopped scallions

¼ cup sliced almonds, toasted

1. Preheat the oven to 400°F. Line a baking sheet with parchment paper.

2. Season the cut sides of the squash with the salt and pepper and drizzle with 1 tablespoon of sesame oil. Place cut-side down on the prepared baking sheet and bake for 35 to 45 minutes, until tender. Set aside to cool.

3. In a small bowl, whisk together the brown sugar substitute, lime juice, and soy sauce until the sugar is dissolved. Stir in the tahini and red pepper flakes. Add the water if the sauce is too thick. Season with salt and pepper to taste.

4. In a large skillet, heat the remaining 1 tablespoon of sesame oil over medium-high heat. Add the edamame, carrots, ginger, and garlic and sauté for 5 to 7 minutes, until the edamame begin to brown and the carrots are tender. Remove from the heat.

5. Using a fork, scrape and scoop out the flesh from the spaghetti squash halves, creating strands. (Keep the spaghetti squash shells for serving.) Stir the squash strands into the vegetable mixture.

6. Divide the squash and edamame mixture between the spaghetti squash shells. Drizzle each serving with the sauce and garnish with the scallions and almonds. Serve with the lime wedges for squeezing.

VARIATION: Give it a Thai twist: Add some chopped fresh mint to the vegetables, use no-sugar-added peanut butter instead of the tahini, and garnish with chopped dry-roasted peanuts instead of sliced almonds.

Per serving: Calories: 500; Total fat: 39g; Saturated Fat: 5g; Total Carbs: 32g; Fiber: 10g; Net Carbs: 22g; Protein: 14g; Sodium: 1,101mg; Sweetener: 12g

Macros: Fat: 66%; Carbs: 24%; Protein: 10%

Vegetable Fajita Bowl with Cilantro-Lime Crema

Gluten-Free, Low-Sodium, Vegetarian

SERVES 2 | PREP TIME: 15 MINUTES | COOK TIME: 10 MINUTES

This is such an easy weeknight meal that you can have on the table within 30 minutes. Also, this recipe is super versatile—use whatever veggies you have on hand at the end of the week when you need to clean out the refrigerator. Sometimes I like to throw a fried egg on top and have it for brunch.

2 tablespoons sour cream

4 tablespoons finely chopped fresh cilantro, divided

2 limes, 1 juiced and 1 cut into wedges

1 tablespoon mayonnaise

Sea salt

Freshly ground black pepper

1 tablespoon avocado oil or extra-virgin olive oil

8 baby bella (cremini) mushrooms, quartered

1 medium zucchini, sliced into ½-inch-thick rounds

4 asparagus spears, trimmed and halved

½ white onion, thinly sliced

1 poblano pepper, thinly sliced

½ teaspoon ground cumin

¼ teaspoon dried oregano

1. In a small bowl, make the crema by whisking together the sour cream, 2 tablespoons cilantro, juice of 1 lime, and the mayonnaise. Season with a pinch of salt and pepper to taste and refrigerate to chill.

2. In a large skillet, heat the oil over medium-high heat. Add the mushrooms, zucchini, asparagus, onion, poblano pepper, cumin, and oregano and sauté for 8 to 10 minutes, until the vegetables become tender and slightly browned. Season with another pinch of salt and pepper to taste.

3. Divide between two bowls. Drizzle each with half the crema and garnish with the remaining 2 tablespoons of cilantro. Serve with the lime wedges.

DIETARY SWAP: For a vegan crema, use vegan sour cream, replace the mayonnaise with avocado oil, and blend in a food processor to create a thick dressing.

Per serving: Calories: 204; Total fat: 15g; Saturated Fat: 3g; Total Carbs: 16g; Fiber: 4g; Net Carbs: 12g; Protein: 5g; Sodium: 148mg; Sweetener: 0g

Macros: Fat: 67%; Carbs: 26%; Protein: 7%

Spinach and Artichoke Pie

Extra Low-Carb, Gluten-Free

SERVES 2 | PREP TIME: 10 MINUTES | COOK TIME: 20 MINUTES

This low-carb version offers the same flavors as my favorite childhood dip but instead it's a pie! This pie crust can be used for other recipes as well, both sweet (just add a teaspoon of sweetener) and savory.

Nonstick cooking spray
2 large eggs, divided
½ tablespoon butter, melted, divided
¾ cup almond flour
¾ teaspoon sea salt, divided

½ tablespoon extra-virgin olive oil or avocado oil
½ white onion, chopped
4 garlic cloves, minced
2 cups chopped spinach
½ cup canned artichoke hearts, drained and chopped

½ cup shredded mozzarella cheese
¼ cup shredded Parmesan cheese
1 scallion, green tops only, chopped
½ teaspoon freshly ground black pepper

1. Preheat the oven to 350°F. Mist a mini loaf pan with cooking spray.

2. In a small bowl, mix together 1 egg and half the butter until well combined. Stir in the almond flour and ¼ teaspoon of salt. Scoop the mixture into the prepared pan, patting it down to fill the pan. Bake for 8 to 10 minutes, until the crust becomes slightly firm.

3. In a small skillet, heat the oil over medium-high heat. Add the onion and garlic and cook for 2 minutes, until the onion is tender. Transfer to a bowl and cool for 5 minutes.

4. In a medium bowl, stir together the cooked onion, spinach, artichoke hearts, mozzarella, Parmesan, and scallion greens. Season with the remaining ½ teaspoon of salt and the pepper. Smooth the mixture over the crust and smooth the top.

5. Bake for 8 to 10 minutes, until the spinach and cheese mixture becomes lightly firm to the touch. Cool for 5 minutes.

6. Cut into 4 slices and serve 2 slices per person.

COOKING TIP: When you pat the crust into the loaf pan, lightly dampen your hands so the batter doesn't stick to them.

Per serving: Calories: 530; Total fat: 38g; Saturated Fat: 10g; Total Carbs: 24g; Fiber: 10g; Net Carbs: 14g; Protein: 26g; Sodium: 1,366mg; Sweetener: 0g

Macros: Fat: 64%; Carbs: 17%; Protein: 19%

Stuffed Acorn Squash

Gluten-Free

SERVES 2 | PREP TIME: 10 MINUTES | COOK TIME: 55 MINUTES

Growing up in a large family, Thanksgiving morning was always so exciting because of that "Thanksgiving smell." I would be the first one out of bed so I could help my parents prepare the feast. This flavorful stuffed acorn squash will have you craving a full-blown Thanksgiving meal.

1 medium acorn squash, halved lengthwise and seeded

2 tablespoons avocado oil or extra-virgin olive oil, divided

1 teaspoon sea salt, divided

1½ teaspoons freshly ground black pepper, divided

1 cup chopped kale

1 cup riced cauliflower

¼ cup chopped pecans

1 tablespoon grated orange zest

1 tablespoon chopped fresh thyme leaves

½ cup shredded Parmesan cheese

2 tablespoons low-sodium vegetable stock

Chopped fresh parsley, for garnish

1. Preheat the oven to 400°F. Line a baking sheet with parchment paper.

2. On the prepared baking sheet, drizzle the squash with 1 tablespoon of oil, ½ teaspoon of salt, and ½ teaspoon of pepper. Place cut-side down and roast for 30 to 40 minutes, until fork-tender. Remove from the oven but leave the oven on.

3. Meanwhile, in a medium skillet, heat the remaining 1 tablespoon of oil over medium-high heat. Add the kale and cauliflower and cook for 5 to 7 minutes, until the cauliflower becomes tender. Add the pecans, orange zest, and thyme and cook for 2 minutes, or until the cauliflower is lightly browned. Remove from the heat and let cool for 5 minutes.

4. Stir in the Parmesan, vegetable stock, and remaining ½ teaspoon of salt and 1 teaspoon of pepper.

5. Flip the squash cut-side up. Divide the stuffing mixture between the squash halves. Cover with aluminum foil and bake for 10 to 12 minutes, until the cheese is melted.

6. Garnish with parsley and enjoy.

DIETARY SWAP: Use 1 to 2 teaspoons of nut butter in place of the Parmesan to make this dairy-free. It will complement the sweet and earthy flavor of the acorn squash wonderfully.

Per serving: Calories: 428; Total fat: 31g; Saturated Fat: 6g; Total Carbs: 31g; Fiber: 6g; Net Carbs: 25g; Protein: 11g; Sodium: 1,359mg; Sweetener: 0g

Macros: Fat: 63%; Carbs: 27%; Protein: 10%

Zucchini, Mushroom, and Spinach White Lasagna

Gluten-Free

SERVES 2 | PREP TIME: 15 MINUTES | COOK TIME: 40 MINUTES

White lasagna is so rich and decadent; it's one of my favorite dishes. Swapping out the carb-loaded pasta for zucchini and mushrooms allows me to enjoy this without guilt. Serve with a big garden salad on the side.

Nonstick cooking spray

1 medium zucchini, cut lengthwise into ¼-inch-thick strips

1 tablespoon avocado oil or extra-virgin olive oil

½ white onion, chopped

½ cup chopped mushrooms

4 garlic cloves, thinly sliced

½ cup ricotta cheese

¼ cup shaved Parmesan cheese

½ cup shredded mozzarella cheese, divided

1 large egg

1 teaspoon sea salt

½ teaspoon ground white pepper

¼ cup half-and-half

2 cups chopped baby spinach

1. Preheat the oven to 350°F. Mist a mini loaf pan with cooking spray.

2. Line a baking sheet with paper towels. In a nonstick skillet, working in batches, cook the zucchini strips over medium-high heat for 1 minute per side. Transfer to the paper towel–lined pan. Continue until all the zucchini strips are cooked.

3. In the same skillet, heat the oil over medium-high heat. Add the onion, mushrooms, and garlic and cook for 7 to 9 minutes, until the onions are tender.

4. In a medium bowl, stir together the ricotta, Parmesan, ¼ cup of mozzarella, the egg, salt, and white pepper.

5. Pour the half-and half into the prepared loaf pan. Add a layer of zucchini, half the cheese mixture, half the chopped spinach, and half the onion and mushroom mixture. Repeat, finishing with zucchini slices on the top. Top with the remaining ¼ cup of mozzarella.

6. Bake for 20 to 30 minutes, until the cheese has melted. Let sit for 5 minutes before cutting into slices and serving.

COOKING TIP: Partially precooking the zucchini helps draw the moisture out so you won't have a waterlogged, runny lasagna—no one's idea of a good time.

Per serving: Calories: 430; Total fat: 31g; Saturated Fat: 15g; Total Carbs: 15g; Fiber: 2g; Net Carbs: 13g; Protein: 24g; Sodium: 1,408mg; Sweetener: 0g

Macros: Fat: 64%; Carbs: 13%; Protein: 23%

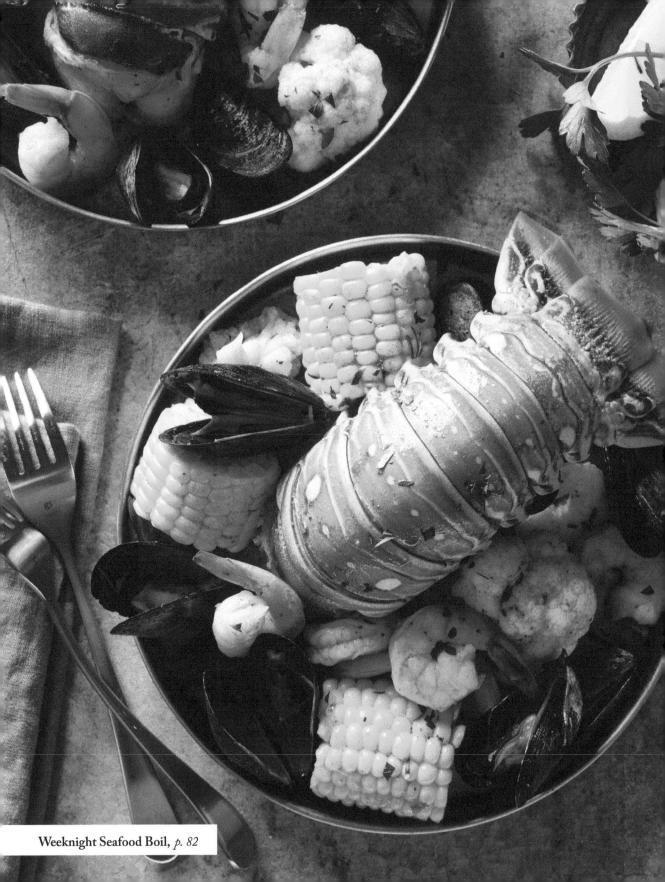

Weeknight Seafood Boil, *p. 82*

Chapter Five

FISH AND SHELLFISH

Green Curry Poached Salmon Bowls

Dairy-Free, Extra Low-Carb, Gluten-Free, Low-Sodium

SERVES 2 | PREP TIME: 15 MINUTES | COOK TIME: 35 MINUTES

Don't let the simplicity of this dish fool you into thinking it lacks flavor. The savory green curry pairs so well with the rich yet delicate taste of salmon. Bonus: Salmon is a powerhouse protein full of healthy omega-3 fats that will keep you fueled for hours.

2 cups low-sodium vegetable stock

1 cup full-fat coconut milk

1 tablespoon Thai green curry paste

2 salmon fillets (5 ounces each), skinned

½ red bell pepper, thinly sliced

½ cup shredded red cabbage

Sea salt

Freshly ground black pepper

2 cups roughly chopped baby spinach

1 lime, halved

2 tablespoons chopped fresh cilantro

1. In a medium saucepan, bring the vegetable stock, coconut milk, and green curry paste to a boil over medium-high heat. Reduce the heat to medium-low.

2. Add the salmon fillets, bell pepper, and cabbage and simmer for 8 to 10 minutes, until the salmon is cooked through. Season with salt and black pepper to taste.

3. Divide the baby spinach between two bowls. Top each with a salmon fillet. Dividing evenly, top with the vegetables and broth.

4. Garnish each bowl with a lime half and cilantro and serve.

VARIATION: Swap the salmon out for cod and simmer for 6 to 8 minutes.

Per serving: Calories: 463; Total fat: 34g; Saturated Fat: 23g; Total Carbs: 11g; Fiber: 4g; Net Carbs: 7g; Protein: 32g; Sodium: 188mg; Sweetener: 0g

Macros: Fat: 62%; Carbs: 9%; Protein: 29%

Sea Scallops with Pesto–White Wine Sauce

Extra Low-Carb, Gluten-Free

SERVES 2 | PREP TIME: 10 MINUTES | COOK TIME: 10 MINUTES

Scallops, pesto, and white wine—a trio that was meant to be! This fresh, light, and flavorful dish is perfect for a hot summer night. The scallops can be swapped out for shrimp or a mild white fish.

8 ounces sea scallops
½ teaspoon sea salt
1 teaspoon freshly ground
  black pepper
2 tablespoons avocado oil
  or extra-virgin olive oil
4 garlic cloves, chopped

½ cup low-sodium
  vegetable stock
¼ cup low-carb dry
  white wine
2 tablespoons pesto
3 cups zoodles
  (spiralized zucchini)

¼ cup grape
  tomatoes, halved
¼ cup thinly sliced
  fresh basil
½ lemon

1. Season the scallops with the salt and pepper.

2. In a large skillet, heat the oil over medium-high heat. Add the scallops and cook on each side for 2 to 3 minutes, until golden brown. Remove from the pan.

3. Set the same pan over medium heat. Add the garlic and sauté for 30 to 45 seconds, until fragrant. Add the vegetable stock and wine and simmer for 2 minutes, stirring and scraping up any bits from the bottom of the pan.

4. Stir in the pesto. Add the zoodles and tomatoes and mix well. Return the scallops to the pan and cover with a lid for 30 seconds to a minute to warm them up.

5. Divide evenly between two bowls. Garnish with fresh basil, squeeze the lemon juice over the dish, and serve.

DIETARY SWAP: Lower the carbs and calories by swapping the white wine for additional vegetable stock.

Per serving: Calories: 329; Total fat: 24g; Saturated Fat: 3g; Total Carbs: 12g; Fiber: 2g; Net Carbs: 10g; Protein: 18g; Sodium: 1,070mg; Sweetener: 0g

Macros: Fat: 64%; Carbs: 15%; Protein: 21%

Cilantro-Lime Shrimp and Peppers

Gluten-Free

SERVES 2 | PREP TIME: 15 MINUTES | COOK TIME: 15 MINUTES

Here's a super-speedy meal that you can have on the table within minutes. What makes this dish sing is the freshly squeezed lime juice and cilantro at the end—so don't skimp on that! I like to serve this with my Chili and Cumin Fried Cauliflower "Rice" (page 112) for a delicious spicy dinner.

2 tablespoon avocado oil or extra-virgin olive oil
1 white onion, thinly sliced
½ green bell pepper, sliced
½ red bell pepper, thinly sliced

2 garlic cloves, thinly sliced
1 pound medium shrimp, peeled and deveined
¼ cup chopped fresh cilantro
Juice of 2 limes

½ teaspoon sea salt
½ teaspoon red pepper flakes
¼ cup crumbled Cotija or feta cheese
1 avocado, sliced

1. In a large skillet, heat the oil over medium-high heat until shimmering. Add the onion, bell peppers, and garlic and stir-fry for 6 to 8 minutes, until the vegetables begin to soften.

2. Add the shrimp to the skillet and cook, tossing with the vegetables, for about 4 minutes, or until the shrimp are pink and firm.

3. Remove from the heat and stir in the cilantro, lime juice, salt, and red pepper flakes.

4. Evenly divide the shrimp and vegetables between two bowls. Top each serving with 2 tablespoons Cotija and half the avocado and serve.

COOKING TIP: Save on prep time by buying frozen shrimp that are already peeled. I like to keep a bag in my freezer at all times for quick meals like this.

Per serving: Calories: 549; Total fat: 35g; Saturated Fat: 8g; Total Carbs: 24g; Fiber: 11g; Net Carbs: 13g; Protein: 52g; Sodium: 1,032mg; Sweetener: 0g

Macros: Fat: 50%; Carbs: 15%; Protein: 35%

Kung Pao Shrimp

Dairy-Free, Extra Low-Carb

SERVES 2 | PREP TIME: 20 MINUTES | COOK TIME: 10 MINUTES

This dinner is easy to whip up any time you get cravings for takeout. If you can't find dried red chiles, substitute ½ teaspoon red pepper flakes or half a fresh jalapeño. This is great served on a bed of spiralized zucchini or riced cauliflower.

2 tablespoons reduced-sodium soy sauce

1 teaspoon brown sugar substitute

½ teaspoon apple cider vinegar

1½ teaspoons minced garlic, divided

1 teaspoon minced peeled fresh ginger, divided

½ teaspoon sesame oil

¼ teaspoon red pepper flakes

1 tablespoon avocado oil or extra-virgin olive oil

8 ounces medium shrimp, peeled and deveined

½ red bell pepper, diced

1 celery stalk, cut into ¼-inch-thick slices

4 dried red chiles, halved and seeded

¼ cup roughly chopped unsalted roasted peanuts

1. In a small bowl, whisk the soy sauce, brown sugar substitute, and vinegar until the sweetener has dissolved. Whisk in 1 teaspoon of garlic, ½ teaspoon of ginger, the sesame oil, and red pepper flakes. Set the sauce aside.

2. In a large nonstick skillet, heat the oil over medium-high heat. Add the shrimp, bell pepper, and celery and cook for 4 minutes, stirring frequently, until the shrimp are pink and cooked through. Add the dried red chiles and the remaining ½ teaspoon of ginger and ½ teaspoon of garlic and cook for an additional minute, until fragrant. Add the sauce and cook for 3 to 4 minutes, stirring frequently, until the sauce is bubbling.

3. Divide between two bowls. Garnish with the peanuts.

VARIATION: Chicken would work in this recipe, too. In step 2, add the chicken and cook for 2 minutes before adding the celery and red bell pepper.

Per serving: Calories: 298; Total fat: 18g; Saturated Fat: 3g; Total Carbs: 10g; Fiber: 2g; Net Carbs: 6g; Protein: 29g; Sodium: 655mg; Sweetener: 2g

Macros: Fat: 53%; Carbs: 11%; Protein: 36%

Beer-Battered Coconut Shrimp with Orange Marmalade

Dairy-Free, Extra Low-Carb

SERVES 2 | PREP TIME: 10 MINUTES | COOK TIME: 10 MINUTES

Having worked many years in the restaurant industry, I've made a lot of beer-battered coconut shrimp. This is my low-carb version that can be served as an entrée, as an appetizer, or with a steak for surf 'n' turf night.

1 cup unsweetened coconut flakes, divided

½ cup low-carb beer

1 large egg

½ cup almond flour

½ teaspoon sea salt

¼ teaspoon baking powder

¼ teaspoon freshly ground black pepper

¼ cup sugar-free orange marmalade

1 teaspoon stone-ground prepared mustard

½ teaspoon prepared horseradish

8 ounces large shrimp, peeled and deveined, tails on

3 tablespoons avocado oil, for frying

1. Place the coconut flakes in a baking dish and cover with a towel to prevent drying out.

2. In a medium bowl, gently whisk together the beer and egg. Whisk in the almond flour, 3 tablespoons of coconut flakes, the salt, baking powder, and pepper. Whisk for 30 seconds to ensure there are no clumps. Set aside.

3. In a small bowl, make the dipping sauce by whisking together the orange marmalade, mustard, and horseradish. Set aside.

4. Line a baking sheet with parchment paper. Grab a shrimp by the tail and gently dip it into the beer batter, allowing the excess batter to drip back off into the bowl. Dip each side of the shrimp into the coconut flakes to evenly coat, then set on the prepared baking sheet. Repeat until all shrimp are coated.

5. Line a plate with paper towels. In a medium skillet, heat the oil over medium-low heat until shimmering. Working in batches, cook the shrimp for 3 to 5 minutes per side, until they are golden brown and crispy. Drain on the paper towels.

6. Serve hot with the dipping sauce.

COOKING TIP: You can also bake these in a 400°F oven. Place the shrimp on a parchment-lined baking sheet and mist them with cooking spray. Bake for 20 minutes, flipping halfway through.

Per serving: Calories: 553; Total fat: 43g; Saturated Fat: 15g; Total Carbs: 13g; Fiber: 7g; Net Carbs: 6g; Protein: 33g; Sodium: 698mg; Sweetener: 0g

Macros: Fat: 67%; Carbs: 23%; Protein: 10%

Sesame Tuna with Garlic Bok Choy

Dairy-Free, Extra Low-Carb

SERVES 2 | PREP TIME: 10 MINUTES | COOK TIME: 10 MINUTES

Sesame seeds make a wonderful crust for fish, especially tuna, because they offer a lovely toasty flavor and a delightful crunch. Tuna is a relatively lean protein that is high in omega-3 fatty acids, which are beneficial for heart health.

½ tablespoon black sesame seeds
½ tablespoon white sesame seeds
Grated zest and juice of 1 lime
2 (6-ounce) tuna steaks

2 tablespoons avocado oil or extra-virgin olive oil, divided
1 head bok choy, quartered lengthwise
6 garlic cloves, thinly sliced

2 tablespoons reduced-sodium soy sauce
1 scallion, chopped

1. In a small bowl, mix together both sesame seeds and the lime zest until combined.

2. Evenly rub the top and bottom of each tuna steak with about ½ tablespoon of oil. Sprinkle the sesame seed mixture onto the top and bottom of each steak and set aside.

3. In a large skillet, heat the remaining 1 tablespoon oil over medium-high heat. Add the tuna and cook for 2 to 5 minutes per side, depending on the desired doneness. Remove and set aside to rest.

4. In the skillet, cook the bok choy, cut-side down, for 1 minute. Flip, add the garlic, and cook for an additional minute. Add the soy sauce and toss to lightly coat the bok choy. Cover and cook for 5 minutes, or until the center of the bok choy is tender.

5. Plate 2 bok choy quarters each on two plates. Top each with a tuna steak. Drizzle with the cooking liquid and lime juice and garnish with the scallion.

COOKING TIP: I think tuna is wonderful medium-rare, so I like to stick to the lower end of the cooking time.

Per serving: Calories: 384; Total fat: 17g; Saturated Fat: 2g; Total Carbs: 11g; Fiber: 3g; Net Carbs: 8g; Protein: 45g; Sodium: 607mg; Sweetener: 0g

Macros: Fat: 40%; Carbs: 10%; Protein: 50%

Squid and Tomato Stew with Olives and Greens

Gluten-Free

SERVES 2 | PREP TIME: 10 MINUTES | COOK TIME: 10 MINUTES

This is a very light, yet flavorful Mediterranean-style stew. If you're unable to get your hands on fresh squid, frozen will work just as well. I love serving it with some riced cauliflower or zoodles—they soak up all that delicious tomato-y goodness.

1 tablespoon extra-virgin olive oil

6 white mushrooms, quartered

½ white onion, minced

4 garlic cloves, thinly sliced

8 ounces squid

1 (14.5-ounce) can stewed tomatoes, undrained

¼ cup green olives, halved

4 cups baby spinach

Sea salt

Freshly ground black pepper

¼ cup crumbled feta cheese

¼ cup chopped fresh basil

1 lemon, halved

1. In a large skillet, heat the oil over medium-high heat. Add the mushrooms, onion, and garlic and cook for 4 minutes, or until the onion is just tender.

2. Stir in the squid, stewed tomatoes and their juices, and the green olives. Cover, reduce the heat to medium-low, and simmer for 5 minutes, or until the squid becomes firm and cooked through. Stir in the baby spinach. Season with salt and pepper to taste.

3. Divide between two bowls and garnish with the feta and basil. Serve with a lemon half for squeezing.

VARIATION: You can alter this simple dish in so many ways. Instead of squid, use shrimp or mussels. Instead of feta, use Parmesan shavings. Instead of basil, use fresh oregano. Make this recipe uniquely yours.

Per serving: Calories: 312; Total fat: 15g; Saturated Fat: 5g; Total Carbs: 21g; Fiber: 7g; Net Carbs: 14g; Protein: 26g; Sodium: 712mg; Sweetener: 0g

Macros: Fat: 42%; Carbs: 25%; Protein: 33%

Parmesan-Baked Tilapia with Creamed Kale

Gluten-Free

SERVES 2 | PREP TIME: 10 MINUTES | COOK TIME: 30 MINUTES

This recipe was my answer to fried fish with gravy, a favorite comfort food from my pre-low-carb days. The crunch of the Parmesan-crusted fish paired with the creaminess of the kale is so satisfying and dreamy.

¼ cup shredded
  Parmesan cheese
¼ cup almond flour
½ teaspoon chopped fresh
  thyme leaves
½ teaspoon sea salt
½ teaspoon freshly ground
  black pepper

1 large egg, beaten
2 tablespoons water
2 bunches kale, stems and
  midribs removed
1 tablespoon extra-virgin
  olive oil
½ white onion, chopped
2 garlic cloves, chopped

½ cup heavy
  (whipping) cream
¼ teaspoon
  ground nutmeg
¼ teaspoon red pepper
  flakes (optional)
2 tilapia fillets
  (5 ounces each)

1. On a plate, mix the Parmesan, almond flour, thyme, salt, and pepper. In a small bowl, mix the egg and water. Set both aside.

2. Fill a medium soup pot halfway with water and bring to a boil. Add the kale and cook for 5 minutes, or until it turns a vibrant green. Remove from the water, allow to slightly cool, and roughly chop. Set aside.

3. In a medium saucepan, heat the oil over medium-high heat. Add the onion and garlic and cook for 3 to 5 minutes, until the onion is just tender. Add the cream, nutmeg, and red pepper flakes (if using). Reduce the heat to medium-low, cover, and cook for an additional 10 minutes, stirring occasionally, to thicken and reduce the sauce. Season with salt and pepper.

4. Preheat the broiler to high. Line a baking sheet with parchment paper.

5. Dip each tilapia fillet into the egg mixture and then evenly coat each side with the almond flour mixture. Set the fillets on the prepared baking sheet and broil for 8 to 9 minutes, until the fish is crispy and cooked through.

6. To serve, divide the creamed kale between two plates and top each with a tilapia fillet.

COOKING TIP: When breading the tilapia, use one hand for the wet batter and the other hand for the dry breading.

Per serving: Calories: 657; Total fat: 45g; Saturated Fat: 19g; Total Carbs: 24g; Fiber: 8g; Net Carbs: 16g; Protein: 47g; Sodium: 888mg; Sweetener: 0g

Macros: Fat: 61%; Carbs: 13%; Protein: 26%

Weeknight Seafood Boil

Dairy-Free, Gluten-Free

SERVES 2 | PREP TIME: 10 MINUTES | COOK TIME: 15 MINUTES

This meal was inspired by my ma. Every time she visited us, she would request that we do a big seafood bake for her. This lazy weeknight version can be on your table in no time. Lobster tails are usually found in the frozen seafood section of most supermarkets, and they're surprisingly economical.

½ cup low-carb dry white wine

½ cup vegetable stock

3 lemons, 2 zested and juiced, 1 cut into wedges

2 tablespoons Cajun seasoning, plus more for garnish

½ head cauliflower, cut into 1-inch pieces

1 ear corn, quartered

8 ounces shell-on medium shrimp

8 ounces mussels

2 lobster tails

¼ cup chopped fresh parsley

1. In a medium soup pot, combine the wine, vegetable stock, zest of 2 lemons, lemon juice, and Cajun seasoning. Cover and bring to a simmer over medium heat.

2. Add the cauliflower and corn. Cover and simmer for 7 to 9 minutes, until the cauliflower is al dente.

3. Add the shrimp, mussels, and lobster tails. Cover and simmer for an additional 5 minutes, or until the seafood is cooked through.

4. Pour into a large serving dish and garnish with parsley, lemon wedges, and additional Cajun seasoning for added spice. (Save the broth for a flavorful base for a soup or stock in the future; store in the freezer.)

DIETARY SWAP: Lower the carbs by replacing the corn with ½-inch slices of zucchini. Add them in the last 2 minutes of cooking.

Per serving: Calories: 355; Total fat: 4g; Saturated Fat: 1g; Total Carbs: 24g; Fiber: 4g; Net Carbs: 20g; Protein: 58g; Sodium: 971mg; Sweetener: 0g

Macros: Fat: 10%; Carbs: 24%; Protein: 66%

Broiled Snapper with Avocado, Grapefruit, and Fennel Slaw

Gluten-Free

SERVES 2 | PREP TIME: 15 MINUTES | COOK TIME: 10 MINUTES

Fresh, light, vibrant, and flavorful is the best way to describe this dish. This is a wonderfully healthy dish that is perfect for a hot summer evening. The sweet versus sour flavor from the grapefruit slaw is the perfect complement to the light and flaky snapper.

- 2 snapper fillets (6 ounces each)
- ½ teaspoon sea salt
- ½ teaspoon freshly ground black pepper
- 1½ tablespoons avocado oil or extra-virgin olive oil, divided
- 1 pink grapefruit, ½ cut into segments and ½ juiced
- 1 small bulb fennel, thinly shaved
- 1 cup baby spinach
- 2 radishes, thinly sliced
- 1 tablespoon thinly sliced fresh basil
- ¼ jalapeño, seeded and minced
- ½ teaspoon apple cider vinegar
- ½ teaspoon granulated sugar substitute
- 2 garlic cloves, minced
- 1 avocado, cubed
- ¼ cup shaved Parmesan cheese

1. Preheat the broiler on high. Line a baking sheet with parchment paper.

2. Arrange the snapper on the prepared baking sheet and season with the salt and pepper. Drizzle with ½ tablespoon of oil. Set aside.

3. In a medium bowl, combine the grapefruit segments and juice, fennel, spinach, radishes, basil, jalapeño, vinegar, sugar substitute, garlic, and the remaining 1 tablespoon of oil. Mix well and refrigerate for 15 minutes.

4. Broil the snapper for 8 to 10 minutes, until cooked through.

5. Divide the chilled fennel slaw between two plates. Top the slaw with a snapper fillet, half the avocado, and 2 tablespoons Parmesan.

DIETARY SWAP: Use salmon in place of the tilapia for more omega-3s.

Per serving: Calories: 582; Total fat: 32g; Saturated Fat: 6g; Total Carbs: 34g; Fiber: 14g; Net Carbs: 20g; Protein: 45g; Sodium: 990mg; Sweetener: 1g

Macros: Fat: 47%; Carbs: 21%; Protein: 32%

Paprika Fish Sticks with Rémoulade Sauce

Dairy-Free, Extra Low-Carb, Gluten-Free

SERVES 2 | PREP TIME: 15 MINUTES | COOK TIME: 12 MINUTES

When I was a kid, we had fish sticks with tartar sauce every Friday night—no questions asked. This is my healthier take on those frozen fish sticks. Paired with my Lobster Moc 'n' Cheese (page 116), this is a grown-up meal I can get behind.

¼ cup mayonnaise
¼ green bell pepper, minced
Juice of ½ lemon
1 tablespoon minced white onion
1 garlic clove, minced

1 teaspoon whole-grain mustard
¾ teaspoon sea salt, divided
½ teaspoon freshly ground black pepper, divided
8 ounces cod fillets, cut into ½-inch-wide slices

1½ teaspoons smoked paprika, divided
1 large egg
1 tablespoon water
½ cup almond flour
Nonstick cooking spray

1. Preheat the oven to 450°F. Set a wire rack in a baking sheet.

2. To make the rémoulade, in a small bowl, mix the mayonnaise, bell pepper, lemon juice, onion, garlic, mustard, ¼ teaspoon of salt, and ¼ teaspoon of pepper.

3. Season the cod with 1 teaspoon smoked paprika and the remaining ½ teaspoon of salt and ¼ teaspoon of pepper.

4. In a small bowl, whisk the egg and water. On a large plate, mix the almond flour and remaining ½ teaspoon smoked paprika.

5. Dip the cod into the egg and then the almond flour and place on the wire rack. Mist the top of the fish with cooking spray.

6. Cook for 10 to 12 minutes, until golden brown.

7. Serve hot with the rémoulade on the side.

Per serving: Calories: 456; Total fat: 36g; Saturated Fat: 5g; Total Carbs: 9g; Fiber: 4g; Net Carbs: 5g; Protein: 26g; Sodium: 1,282mg; Sweetener: 0g

Macros: Fat: 69%; Carbs: 7%; Protein: 24%

Crispy-Skin Salmon with Roasted Ratatouille

Gluten-Free

SERVES 2 | PREP TIME: 10 MINUTES | COOK TIME: 10 MINUTES

I have a friend who eats salmon, including the skin, at almost every meal. If you have not tried crispy salmon skin, you're totally missing out—it is delicious! Salmon is not only extremely nutritious, but also amazing for your hair, skin, and nails.

1 medium zucchini, cut into ½-inch cubes

2 Roma (plum) tomatoes, cut into ½-inch-thick slices

1 Japanese eggplant, cut into ½-inch cubes

½ orange bell pepper, cut into ½-inch chunks

¼ red onion, thinly sliced

3 garlic cloves, thinly sliced

6 thyme sprigs, leaves picked

1½ tablespoons avocado oil, divided

2 teaspoons sea salt, divided

1 teaspoon freshly ground black pepper, divided

2 salmon fillets (4 ounces each)

¼ cup grated Parmesan cheese

1. Preheat the oven to 400°F.

2. On a baking sheet, toss the zucchini, tomatoes, eggplant, bell pepper, red onion, garlic, thyme leaves, ½ tablespoon of oil, 1 teaspoon of salt, and ½ teaspoon of pepper.

3. Cover with aluminum foil and bake for 30 minutes. Uncover and bake for an additional 10 minutes, or until the vegetables are tender.

4. Meanwhile, season both sides of the salmon with the remaining 1 teaspoon of salt and ½ teaspoon of pepper.

5. In a medium skillet, heat the remaining 1 tablespoon of oil over medium-high heat. Cook the salmon, skin-side down, for 5 minutes. Flip and cook for an additional 2 to 5 minutes, until firm and flakes with a fork.

6. Divide the ratatouille and salmon between two plates. Garnish with the Parmesan.

COOKING TIP: The more you salt the skin side of the salmon, the crispier it will become, so if sodium is not an issue for you, salt generously!

Per serving: Calories: 377; Total fat: 22g; Saturated Fat: 4g; Total Carbs: 17g; Fiber: 5g; Net Carbs: 12g; Protein: 29g; Sodium: 2,034mg; Sweetener: 0g

Macros: Fat: 52%; Carbs: 16%; Protein: 32%

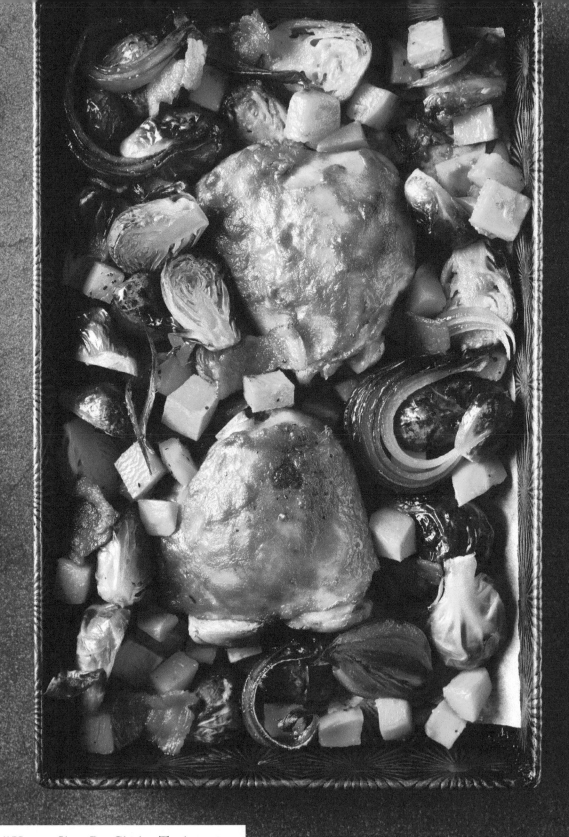

Fall Harvest Sheet Pan Chicken Thighs, *p. 91*

Chapter Six

POULTRY AND MEAT

Turkey Tenderloin with Lemon-Dijon Artichoke Sauce

Extra Low-Carb, Gluten-Free

SERVES 2 | PREP TIME: 10 MINUTES | COOK TIME: 15 MINUTES

I love turkey tenderloin because it's so easy to cook and it stays so moist. When it's paired with a vibrant sauce like this one, you just can't beat it for an easy weeknight meal. When purchasing a turkey tenderloin, I typically use only half and freeze the rest for another day.

8 ounces turkey tenderloin, cut into 1-inch pieces

1 teaspoon sea salt, plus more to taste

1½ teaspoons freshly ground black pepper, plus more to taste

1 tablespoon avocado oil or extra-virgin olive oil

½ red bell pepper, diced

¼ cup low-carb dry white wine or chicken broth

4 garlic cloves, chopped

¼ cup roughly chopped canned or thawed frozen artichoke hearts

¼ cup heavy (whipping) cream

1 tablespoon Dijon mustard

½ tablespoon fresh thyme leaves

Juice of ½ lemon

2 tablespoons chopped fresh parsley

1. Season the turkey with salt and black pepper.

2. In a large skillet, heat the oil over medium-high heat. Add the turkey and cook for 3 minutes on each side, until slightly browned. Add the bell pepper and cook for 1 minute, or until it starts to soften.

3. Reduce the heat to medium-low and add the wine and garlic. Using a wooden spoon or spatula, scrape up all the bits on the bottom of the pan. Add the artichoke hearts, cream, mustard, and thyme. Simmer for 5 to 7 minutes, stirring, until the sauce starts to thicken. Add the lemon juice and season with more salt and black pepper.

4. Divide the turkey and vegetables between two plates. Garnish with parsley and serve.

DIETARY SWAP: Replace the heavy cream with half-and-half to lower the fat in this dish. You will need to simmer it a little longer, for 7 to 9 minutes.

Per serving: Calories: 327; Total fat: 21g; Saturated Fat: 8g; Total Carbs: 8g; Fiber: 2g; Net Carbs: 6g; Protein: 28g; Sodium: 1,123mg; Sweetener: 0g

Macros: Fat: 55%; Carbs: 9%; Protein: 36%

Bacon-Wrapped Apricot and Walnut Stuffed Turkey Breast

Extra Low-Carb, Dairy-Free, Gluten-Free

SERVES 2 TO 4 | PREP TIME: 10 MINUTES | COOK TIME: 45 MINUTES

Roasting a whole turkey is overkill for two, which is why I love that you can just roast a turkey breast instead. Wrapping this stuffed turkey breast with bacon adds even more flavor and juiciness.

1 tablespoon avocado oil
 or extra-virgin olive oil
½ white onion, diced
¼ cup walnuts
3 fresh apricots, pitted

2 tablespoons chopped
 fresh parsley
2 teaspoons chopped
 fresh rosemary
1 teaspoon sea salt, divided

¾ teaspoon freshly ground
 black pepper, divided
½ (3-pound) turkey
 breast, butterflied
4 bacon slices

1. Preheat the oven to 350°F.

2. In an ovenproof medium skillet, heat the oil over medium-high heat. Add the onion and sauté for 5 minutes, or until just browned.

3. In a food processor, pulse the walnuts, apricots, parsley, and rosemary until well combined. Add the sautéed onion and pulse again to incorporate. Season with ½ teaspoon of salt and ¼ teaspoon of pepper. (Set the ovenproof skillet aside.)

4. Season the turkey breast with the remaining ½ teaspoon of salt and ½ teaspoon of pepper on both sides.

5. Spread the stuffing onto one side of the breast and close. Starting at the narrow end of the breast, tightly wrap the bacon slices around the turkey breast, working toward the thicker end of the breast. Place in the ovenproof skillet.

6. Transfer the skillet to the oven and bake for 20 minutes. Flip and bake for an additional 20 minutes, until cooked through and the juices run clear.

7. Remove from the oven, cover with foil, and allow to rest for 10 minutes prior to carving.

VARIATION: I like to vary up the fruit in the stuffing. Can't find fresh apricots? Try peaches instead, or even green apple.

Per serving: Calories: 409; Total fat: 24g; Saturated Fat: 5g; Total Carbs: 5g; Fiber: 1g; Net Carbs: 4g; Protein: 42g; Sodium: 716mg; Sweetener: 0g

Macros: Fat: 52%; Carbs: 5%; Protein: 43%

Cheesy Pico de Gallo Chicken Cutlets

Extra Low-Carb, Gluten-Free

SERVES 2 | PREP TIME: 10 MINUTES | COOK TIME: 10 MINUTES

Homemade pico de gallo is a staple in my refrigerator during the summer months because my garden is always bursting with cilantro, tomatoes, and jalapeños and I'm always looking for something to do with them. This chicken, topped with homemade pico and smothered in melted cheese, is a surefire hit with my husband.

2 Roma (plum) tomatoes, diced

¼ white onion, diced

¼ cup chopped fresh cilantro, plus more for garnish

½ jalapeño, seeded and minced

Juice of 2 limes, plus lime wedges for serving

2 chicken cutlets (5 ounces each)

1 tablespoon chili powder

1 teaspoon freshly ground black pepper

½ tablespoon ground cumin

½ teaspoon sea salt

1½ tablespoons avocado oil or extra-virgin olive oil

½ cup shredded pepper Jack cheese

2 tablespoons sour cream

1. Preheat the broiler.

2. In a medium glass or nonreactive bowl, mix the tomatoes, onion, cilantro, jalapeño, and lime juice until well combined. Cover and refrigerate.

3. Season the chicken with the chili powder, pepper, cumin, and salt.

4. In a broilerproof skillet, heat the oil over medium heat. Add the chicken and cook on each side for 5 to 7 minutes, until the juices run clear. Remove from the heat.

5. Top each cutlet with half the pico de gallo and ¼ cup pepper Jack. Run under the broiler for 1 to 2 minutes, until the cheese is melted and browned.

6. Garnish each cutlet with sour cream and cilantro. Serve with lime wedges for squeezing.

COOKING TIP: Because of the acid from the lime juice and tomatoes, you should use only a nonreactive (stainless steel or glass) bowl for the pico de gallo.

Per serving: Calories: 447; Total fat: 27g; Saturated Fat: 9g; Total Carbs: 13g; Fiber: 4g; Net Carbs: 9g; Protein: 38g; Sodium: 872mg; Sweetener: 0g

Macros: Fat: 54%; Carbs: 12%; Protein: 34%

Fall Harvest Sheet Pan Chicken Thighs

Dairy-Free, Extra Low-Carb, Gluten-Free

SERVES 2 | PREP TIME: 10 MINUTES, PLUS 1 HOUR TO MARINATE |
COOK TIME: 25 MINUTES

These marinated chicken thighs are bursting with flavor and almost impossible to over-cook. The longer you marinate the chicken, the better this dish is, so get these marinating before you go to bed and cook them up the next day for dinner.

2 tablespoons avocado oil or extra-virgin olive oil, plus 2 teaspoons

2 tablespoons Dijon mustard

1½ tablespoons balsamic vinegar

2 teaspoons chopped fresh thyme leaves

1½ teaspoons sea salt, divided

1 teaspoon freshly ground black pepper, divided

2 bone-in, skin-on chicken thighs (5 ounces each)

2 cups halved Brussels sprouts

½ cup ½-inch cubes sweet potato

½ red onion, cut into ¼-inch-thick slices

4 bacon slices, chopped

1. In a plastic zip-top bag, mix 2 tablespoons of oil, the mustard, vinegar, thyme, ½ teaspoon of salt, and ½ teaspoon of pepper. Add the chicken and refrigerate for at least 1 hour.

2. Preheat the oven to 425°F. Line a baking sheet with parchment paper.

3. Arrange the Brussels sprouts, sweet potato, red onion, and bacon on the prepared baking sheet. Toss with the remaining 2 teaspoons of oil, 1 teaspoon of salt, and ½ teaspoon of pepper. Mix with your hands to evenly coat the vegetables. Reserving the marinade, nestle the chicken thighs between the vegetables, then pour the reserved marinade over the chicken and vegetables.

4. Bake for 20 to 25 minutes, until the chicken's juices run clear and the vegetables are tender and browned.

5. Divide the vegetables evenly between two plates and top each with a chicken thigh.

Per serving: Calories: 492; Total fat: 35g; Saturated Fat: 9g; Total Carbs: 11g; Fiber: 4g; Net Carbs: 7g; Protein: 33g; Sodium: 1,077mg; Sweetener: 0g

Macros: Fat: 65%; Carbs: 8%; Protein: 27%

Nashville Hot Chicken Tenders and Slaw

Gluten-Free

SERVES 2 | PREP TIME: 20 MINUTES | COOK TIME: 10 MINUTES

Being a Nashville gal, I had to include my healthier, not-fried version of Nashville hot chicken in this book. Nashville hot chicken is a little sweet and a lot spicy, and full of flavor. The creamy coleslaw will help keep your tongue from tingling too much.

10 ounces chicken tenders
2 tablespoons Nashville Hot Chicken Seasoning (page 140), divided
3 tablespoons avocado oil or extra-virgin olive oil, divided
⅓ cup mayonnaise
1 tablespoon heavy (whipping) cream

1 teaspoon apple cider vinegar
2 garlic cloves, minced
½ teaspoon sea salt, plus more to taste
½ teaspoon freshly ground black pepper, plus more to taste
½ head green cabbage, finely sliced

¼ head red cabbage, finely sliced
Hamburger dill pickles, for serving

1. In a medium bowl, combine the chicken tenders, 1 tablespoon of chicken seasoning, and 1 tablespoon of oil. Set aside to marinate.

2. In a small bowl, mix together 1 tablespoon of oil and the remaining 1 tablespoon of chicken seasoning. Set aside.

3. In another medium bowl, stir together the mayonnaise, cream, vinegar, garlic, salt, and pepper. Add both cabbages and mix until well incorporated. Season with more salt and pepper to taste. Refrigerate for at least 15 minutes.

4. In a medium skillet, heat the remaining 1 tablespoon of oil over medium heat until shimmering. Add the chicken tenders and cook for 4 minutes per side, or until the juices run clear and the chicken is cooked through.

5. Divide the coleslaw and chicken between two plates. Drizzle the seasoned oil over the chicken and top with hamburger dill pickles.

Per serving: Calories: 692; Total fat: 53g; Saturated Fat: 9g; Total Carbs: 24g; Fiber: 6g; Net Carbs: 12g; Protein: 37g; Sodium: 1,052mg; Sweetener: 6g

Macros: Fat: 69%; Carbs: 9%; Protein: 22%

Strip Steak with Creamy Peppercorn Sauce

Extra Low-Carb, Gluten-Free

SERVES 2 | PREP TIME: 10 MINUTES | COOK TIME: 15 MINUTES

This recipe is all about this amazing creamy peppercorn sauce that is simple to prepare and full of flavor. This classic sauce can be used on any steak, chicken, or white fish. Add a side of sautéed mushrooms and onions to this recipe to replicate the full steakhouse experience.

1 (10-ounce) strip steak

1 teaspoon sea salt, plus more to taste

1 teaspoon freshly ground black pepper

1 tablespoon avocado oil or extra-virgin olive oil

1 tablespoon minced white onion

1 garlic clove, minced

⅓ cup beef stock

2 tablespoons low-carb white wine (optional)

¼ cup heavy (whipping) cream

½ tablespoon coarsely cracked black pepper

1 teaspoon chopped fresh thyme leaves

½ teaspoon Worcestershire sauce

1 tablespoon chopped fresh parsley

1. Season the steak with the salt and pepper.

2. In a large skillet, heat the oil over medium-high heat. Add the steak and cook for 3 to 5 minutes per side, until the desired doneness is reached. Set aside on a plate.

3. Add the onion and garlic to the skillet and cook for 1 minute, or until fragrant.

4. Reduce the heat to medium-low. Add the beef stock and wine (if using), scraping up the cooked bits on the bottom of the pan. Add the cream, cracked pepper, thyme, and Worcestershire sauce. Simmer for 3 minutes, or until the sauce just begins to thicken. Season with more salt to taste.

5. Slice the steak across the grain into ¼-inch-thick slices. Divide between two plates, drizzle with the peppercorn sauce, and garnish with parsley.

DIETARY SWAP: To cut down some on fat, replace the heavy cream with half-and-half.

Per serving: Calories: 487; Total fat: 41g; Saturated Fat: 17g; Total Carbs: 2g; Fiber: 0g; Net Carbs: 2g; Protein: 27g; Sodium: 1,283mg; Sweetener: 0g

Macros: Fat: 76%; Carbs: 1%; Protein: 23%

Swedish Meatballs

Extra Low-Carb

SERVES 2 | PREP TIME: 15 MINUTES | COOK TIME: 15 MINUTES

The allspice and nutmeg give these Swedish meatballs a delightfully warm and earthy flavor. Finished with a savory cream sauce, this is the ideal comfort food. I often serve this dish over a bed of spiralized zucchini.

2 teaspoons avocado oil or extra-virgin olive oil

¼ white onion, diced

4 ounces ground beef

4 ounces ground pork

¼ cup almond flour

1 large egg

2 tablespoons chopped fresh parsley, plus more for serving

1 garlic clove, minced

½ teaspoon sea salt

½ teaspoon ground white pepper

½ teaspoon freshly ground black pepper

½ teaspoon ground allspice

½ teaspoon ground nutmeg

¾ cup heavy (whipping) cream

2 teaspoons Worcestershire sauce

1 teaspoon reduced-sodium soy sauce

1. In a medium skillet, heat the oil over medium-high heat. Add the onion and cook for 3 minutes, or until just tender. Remove from the heat and cool for 5 minutes.

2. In a medium bowl, mix the onion, beef, pork, almond flour, egg, parsley, garlic, salt, white pepper, black pepper, allspice, and nutmeg until well combined. Divide the mixture into 6 equal portions and roll into meatballs.

3. In the same skillet, cook the meatballs over medium heat for 8 to 10 minutes, turning constantly so they do not burn, until evenly browned on all sides. Spoon off excess grease.

4. Reduce the heat to low and stir in the cream, Worcestershire sauce, and soy sauce. Using a wooden spoon or spatula, scrape up all the bits on the bottom of the pan. Cover and simmer for an additional 5 minutes, or until the meatballs are cooked through.

5. Divide the meatballs and sauce evenly between two plates. Garnish with parsley and serve immediately.

COOKING TIP: After adding the ingredients for the sauce, don't forget to stir and scrape up all the browned bits at the bottom of the pan. That's where all the flavor is.

Per serving: Calories: 695; Total fat: 61g; Saturated Fat: 28g; Total Carbs: 9g; Fiber: 2g; Net Carbs: 7g; Protein: 30g; Sodium: 745mg; Sweetener: 0g

Macros: Fat: 77%; Carbs: 5%; Protein: 18%

Beef and Spinach Stroganoff

Extra Low-Carb, Gluten-Free

SERVES 2 | PREP TIME: 10 MINUTES | COOK TIME: 10 MINUTES

I grew up eating a lot of beef stroganoff over egg noodles. Just by omitting the flour usually used to thicken the sauce, this recipe became low-carb. Serve this over a bed of mashed cauliflower or Shredded Cabbage Noodles (page 138), and you won't even be thinking about those egg noodles.

- 8 ounces sirloin steak, cut into ½-inch-thick slices
- 1 teaspoon sea salt
- 1 teaspoon freshly ground black pepper
- 1 tablespoon avocado oil or extra-virgin olive oil
- 1 cup sliced white mushrooms
- ½ white onion, thinly sliced
- 2 garlic cloves, thinly sliced
- ¼ cup low-carb dry white wine
- ½ cup half-and-half
- ¼ cup sour cream
- 1 teaspoon smoked paprika, plus more for serving
- 4 cups baby spinach
- 2 tablespoons chopped fresh parsley

1. Season the sirloin with the salt and pepper.

2. In a medium skillet, heat the oil over medium heat. Add the beef slices and cook for about 5 minutes, flipping halfway through, or until they start to brown. Transfer to a plate and set aside.

3. In the same skillet, cook the mushrooms, onion, and garlic for 5 minutes, or until the onions begin to turn translucent. Add the wine and simmer for 2 minutes.

4. Return the beef and any juices to the skillet and reduce the heat to medium-low. Add the half-and-half, sour cream, and paprika and simmer for 8 to 10 minutes, until the sauce has thickened and the sirloin is fork-tender.

5. Divide the spinach between two bowls and serve the beef and gravy on top. Garnish with parsley and a sprinkling of smoked paprika.

DIETARY SWAP: Replace the white wine with beef broth to make it lower calorie and even lower in carbs.

Per serving: Calories: 448; Total fat: 32g; Saturated Fat: 13g; Total Carbs: 10g; Fiber: 3g; Net Carbs: 7g; Protein: 29g; Sodium: 948mg; Sweetener: 0g

Macros: Fat: 65%; Carbs: 8%; Protein: 27%

Homemade Italian Sausage with Red Wine and Tomato Sauce

Dairy-Free, Extra Low-Carb, Gluten-Free

SERVES 2 | PREP TIME: 15 MINUTES | COOK TIME: 35 MINUTES

I have always struggled with finding a low-sodium and no-sugar-added sausage at my local supermarkets—so I created my own recipe! Make extra patties and freeze them for a convenient meal. Cook them from frozen in a covered pan over medium-low heat with 1 teaspoon of oil for 10 to 12 minutes, flipping once halfway through.

8 ounces ground pork

1 tablespoon Italian
    Seasoning (page 141)

½ teaspoon extra-virgin
    olive oil

½ red bell pepper, sliced

¼ white onion, sliced

3 garlic cloves, slivered

2 Roma (plum) tomatoes,
    chopped

¼ cup low-carb red wine

½ teaspoon sea salt

½ teaspoon freshly ground
    black pepper

1. In a medium bowl, mix together the ground pork and Italian seasoning until well incorporated. Divide the mixture into 2 equal portions and form into patties about 1 inch thick.

2. In a skillet, heat the olive oil over medium heat. Add the sausage patties, bell pepper, onion, and garlic and cook for about 8 minutes, or until the sausage is browned on both sides, flipping the sausage halfway through.

3. Add the tomatoes, red wine, salt, and black pepper. Cover, reduce the heat to low, and cook for an additional 7 minutes, or until the sausage is cooked through.

4. Serve 1 sausage patty person, topped with the tomato sauce.

DIETARY SWAP: For a lower-fat dish, swap the pork for ground chicken, ground turkey, or even ground shrimp.

Per serving: Calories: 356; Total fat: 25g; Saturated Fat: 9g; Total Carbs: 9g; Fiber: 2g; Net Carbs: 7g; Protein: 21g; Sodium: 539mg; Sweetener: 0g

Macros: Fat: 66%; Carbs: 9%; Protein: 25%

Black and Blue Pizza with Balsamic and Arugula

Gluten-Free

SERVES 2 | PREP TIME: 10 MINUTES | COOK TIME: 15 MINUTES

This is my favorite salad transformed into a pizza. Steak, blue cheese, and sweet balsamic vinegar are a trio that play so well together. And it's topped with the arugula, so you don't even need to serve this tasty pizza with a salad.

"Fathead" Pizza Crust (page 137)
4 ounces sirloin steak
½ teaspoon sea salt
½ teaspoon freshly ground black pepper, plus more for serving

¼ cup balsamic vinegar
1 tablespoon avocado oil or extra-virgin olive oil
½ red onion, thinly sliced
½ cup shredded Monterey Jack cheese

¼ cup blue cheese crumbles
1 Roma tomato, sliced
2 cups arugula
¼ cup shaved Parmesan cheese

1. Assemble and bake the pizza crust as directed. Leave the oven on and increase the oven temperature to 450°F.

2. Meanwhile, season the steak with the salt and pepper.

3. In a small microwave-safe bowl, microwave the vinegar on high for 3 to 4 minutes, until it has reduced by almost half. Set the balsamic glaze aside to cool.

4. In a medium skillet, heat the oil over medium-high heat. Add the onion and cook for 2 minutes. Remove from the skillet to cool. Add the steak to the pan and cook for 5 minutes per side. Remove from the skillet and let rest for 5 minutes before slicing.

5. Evenly spread the Monterey Jack, blue cheese, tomatoes, and sliced steak over the baked pizza crust. Return to the oven and bake for 8 to 10 minutes, until the cheese is melted and bubbling.

6. Top the pizza with the arugula and Parmesan and season with pepper. Drizzle with the balsamic glaze. Cut into 4 slices and serve 2 slices per person.

VARIATION: Feel free to replace the steak with chicken breast. Add it to the pan after cooking the oil and cook for 8 minutes per side, or until cooked through, then slice before adding to the pizza.

Per serving: Calories: 691; Total fat: 51g; Saturated Fat: 22g; Total Carbs: 16g; Fiber: 3g; Net Carbs: 13g; Protein: 42g; Sodium: 1,453mg; Sweetener: 0g

Macros: Fat: 66%; Carbs: 10%; Protein: 24%

Tarragon and Tomato Smothered Pork Chops

Extra Low-Carb, Gluten-Free

SERVES 2 | PREP TIME: 10 MINUTES PLUS 30 MINUTES TO REST |
COOK TIME: 15 MINUTES

Smothered pork chops served over rice is definitely a Southern favorite! Here's my healthier take with an added burst of flavor from the fresh herbs and lemon. Serve it with riced cauliflower to keep this meal low-carb.

- 2 boneless pork chops (5 ounces each)
- ½ teaspoon sea salt
- ½ teaspoon freshly ground black pepper
- 2 tablespoons avocado oil or extra-virgin olive oil, divided
- ¼ white onion, thinly sliced
- 2 garlic cloves, thinly sliced
- ¼ cup dry white wine
- ¼ cup heavy (whipping) cream
- 2 tablespoons chopped oil-packed sun-dried tomatoes
- 1 tablespoon chopped fresh tarragon
- ½ lemon
- 2 tablespoons chopped fresh parsley

1. Season the pork chops with the salt and pepper and drizzle with 1 tablespoon of oil. Let rest at room temperature for 30 minutes.

2. In a medium skillet, heat the remaining 1 tablespoon of oil over medium-high heat for 30 seconds. Add the pork chops and cook for 4 to 5 minutes per side.

3. Add the onion and garlic and cook for 2 minutes. Reduce the heat to medium-low, add the white wine, and deglaze, stirring to scrape up the browned bits from the bottom, for 30 seconds. Add the cream, sun-dried tomatoes, and tarragon and simmer for 3 to 5 minutes, until the sauce has slightly thickened.

4. Finish by squeezing the lemon juice over the pan and garnish with parsley. Plate one pork chop per person and top with the sauce.

VARIATION: For a twist, add 1 cup sliced red bell peppers and ½ cup sliced white mushrooms along with the onions and garlic. Omit the sun-dried tomatoes and swap the tarragon for fresh oregano.

Per serving: Calories: 470; Total fat: 35g; Saturated Fat: 12g; Total Carbs: 6g; Fiber: 1g; Net Carbs: 5g; Protein: 32g; Sodium: 557mg; Sweetener: 0g

Macros: Fat: 66%; Carbs: 5%; Protein: 29%

Spiced Pork Tenderloin with Sautéed Cabbage and Apples

Dairy-Free, Gluten-Free

SERVES 2 | PREP TIME: 10 MINUTES | COOK TIME: 20 MINUTES

This flavorful spiced pork tenderloin pairs perfectly with the fall flavors of sautéed cabbage and apples. Cutting the pork tenderloin into medallions also makes this recipe speedy, which is wonderful for busy weeknights—I know this dish will become part of your regular rotation.

10 ounces pork tenderloin, cut into ½-inch-thick medallions

1 teaspoon ground allspice

½ teaspoon sea salt

½ teaspoon freshly ground black pepper

2 tablespoons avocado oil or extra-virgin olive oil, divided

¼ red onion, thinly sliced

2 garlic cloves, chopped

½ head green cabbage, thinly sliced

1 Gala apple, thinly sliced

3 thyme sprigs, leaves picked

1 fresh sage leave, chopped

Stone-ground mustard, for serving

1. Season the pork tenderloin with the allspice, salt, and pepper, then rub with 1 tablespoon of oil.

2. In a medium skillet, heat the remaining 1 tablespoon of oil over medium-high heat for 30 seconds. Add the pork medallions and cook for 3 minutes per side. Transfer to a plate to rest.

3. Add the red onion and garlic to the skillet and cook for 1 minute. Add the cabbage, apple, thyme leaves (reserve some for garnish), sage, and the plate drippings from the pork medallions and cook for 10 to 15 minutes, until the cabbage and apples are tender and lightly browned.

4. Make a bed of cabbage and apples each on two plates. Top with the pork medallions and garnish with additional thyme. Serve with mustard on the side.

DIETARY SWAP: To make this even lower in carbs, swap the apple for another half a red onion instead.

Per serving: Calories: 396; Total fat: 19g; Saturated Fat: 3g; Total Carbs: 25g; Fiber: 7g; Net Carbs: 18g; Protein: 32g; Sodium: 573mg; Sweetener: 0g

Macros: Fat: 44%; Carbs: 23%; Protein: 33%

Caribbean Pork Steaks with Mango Salsa

Dairy-Free, Gluten-Free

SERVES 2 | PREP TIME: 15 MINUTES, PLUS 15 MINUTES TO CHILL | COOK TIME: 10 MINUTES

This recipe will have you dreaming of sitting on an island beach. All the wonderful warm spices in this recipe so perfectly complement the sweet and spicy mango salsa. This Caribbean-inspired salsa and rub also work very well with fish.

- 2 Boston butt pork steaks, ½ inch thick (5 ounces each)
- 1 tablespoon avocado oil or extra-virgin olive oil
- 1½ teaspoons sea salt, divided
- 1¼ teaspoons freshly ground black pepper, divided
- 1 teaspoon ground allspice
- 1 teaspoon ground cumin
- 1 teaspoon brown sugar substitute
- 1 mango, diced
- ¼ red bell pepper, diced
- ¼ red onion, minced
- ½ jalapeño, seeded and minced
- Juice of 1 lime
- 2 teaspoons chopped fresh thyme leaves

1. Preheat a gas or charcoal grill. Rub the pork steaks with the oil and season with 1 teaspoon of salt, 1 teaspoon of black pepper, the allspice, cumin, and brown sugar substitute.

2. In a small bowl, combine the mango, bell pepper, red onion, jalapeño, lime juice, and thyme and mix well. Season with the remaining ½ teaspoon of salt and ¼ teaspoon of pepper and place in the refrigerator for at least 15 minutes.

3. Set the pork steaks on the grill grates over the direct heat and cook for 5 minutes per side, until a minimum temperature of 145°F is reached.

4. Serve each pork steak topped with the chilled mango salsa.

COOKING TIP: These pork steaks can also be cooked on the stovetop. In a large skillet, heat 1 tablespoon avocado oil over medium-high heat. Cook the steaks for about 5 minutes per side, until an internal temperature of 145°F is reached.

Per serving: Calories: 450; Total fat: 26g; Saturated Fat: 7g; Total Carbs: 31g; Fiber: 4g; Net Carbs: 27g; Protein: 27g; Sodium: 1,255mg; Sweetener: 2g

Macros: Fat: 51%; Carbs: 24%; Protein: 25%

Coffee-Rubbed Filet Mignon with Blue Cheese and Rosemary Butter

Extra Low-Carb, Gluten-Free

SERVES 2 | PREP TIME: 15 MINUTES | COOK TIME: 10 MINUTES

The reason steakhouse steaks are always so delicious is that they are seasoned well, cooked at a high heat, and finished in butter. Luckily, all are easy to accomplish at home—and you can level up with a fancy compound butter that's deceptively easy to make.

2 tablespoons butter, at room temperature

½ tablespoon crumbled blue cheese

1 garlic clove, minced

½ teaspoon minced fresh rosemary

Juice of ¼ lemon

2 filet mignon steaks (6 ounces each)

2 tablespoons finely ground coffee

½ teaspoon sea salt

½ teaspoon freshly ground black pepper

1 tablespoon avocado oil or extra-virgin olive oil, plus more for drizzling

1. In a small bowl, mash together the butter, blue cheese, garlic, rosemary, and lemon juice with a fork until smooth. Refrigerate to chill.

2. Season the filets with the coffee, salt, pepper, and a drizzle of oil. Set aside.

3. In a large skillet, heat 1 tablespoon of oil over medium-high heat. Add the steaks and cook for 3 to 5 minutes per side, until desired doneness is reached.

4. Serve each steak with a generous 1 tablespoon of the compound butter.

COOKING TIP: I like to make this compound butter in larger quantities to have on hand for flavoring everything from roast chicken to sautéed veggies. Put the butter mixture in some parchment paper and roll it up into a log to keep in the refrigerator.

Per serving: Calories: 598; Total fat: 50g; Saturated Fat: 21g; Total Carbs: 1g; Fiber: 0g; Net Carbs: 1g; Protein: 34g; Sodium: 665mg; Sweetener: 0g

Macros: Fat: 75%; Carbs: 1%; Protein: 24%

Balsamic and Rosemary Rib Eye with Asparagus

Extra Low-Carb, Gluten-Free

SERVES 2 | PREP TIME: 10 MINUTES, PLUS 1 HOUR TO MARINATE | COOK TIME: 15 MINUTES

This wonderful steak dinner will make you think you're eating at a high-end restaurant instead of at home. Add a side of mashed cauliflower and you've got a classic rib-sticking meal.

4 tablespoons avocado oil or extra-virgin olive oil, divided

2 tablespoons balsamic vinegar

2 tablespoons chopped fresh rosemary

1 teaspoon stone-ground mustard

3 garlic cloves, chopped

1 teaspoon sea salt, divided

1 teaspoon freshly ground black pepper, divided

2 rib-eye steaks (5 ounces each)

8 ounces asparagus, trimmed

⅓ cup beef stock

2 tablespoons cold butter

2 tablespoons chopped fresh parsley

1. In a zip-top plastic bag, combine 3 tablespoons of oil, the vinegar, rosemary, mustard, garlic, ½ teaspoon of sea salt, and ½ teaspoon of pepper and mix well. Add the steaks and seal the bag, removing as much air as possible. Refrigerate for at least 1 hour.

2. In a large skillet, heat the remaining 1 tablespoon of oil over medium-high heat. Cook the steaks for 3 to 5 minutes per side, until the desired doneness is reached. Remove from the skillet and let rest for 5 minutes.

3. In the same skillet, toss the asparagus with the remaining ½ teaspoon of salt and ½ teaspoon of pepper. Cook, stirring, for 5 to 7 minutes, until knife-tender. Remove from the skillet and set aside.

4. Pour the beef stock into the skillet to deglaze the pan, stirring to scrape up the browned bits from the bottom. Add the butter and stir constantly until it is melted and well incorporated.

5. Divide the asparagus between two plates and set a steak on each. Drizzle the pan sauce over the steaks and garnish with the parsley.

COOKING TIP: I prefer to marinate my steaks for at least 12 hours to intensify the flavor, so I'll marinate them in the morning before work and cook them up for dinner. Easy-peasy!

Per serving: Calories: 460; Total fat: 36g; Saturated Fat: 14g; Total Carbs: 7g; Fiber: 3g; Net Carbs: 4g; Protein: 31g; Sodium: 796mg; Sweetener: 0g

Macros: Fat: 71%; Carbs: 4%; Protein: 25%

Red Wine Chuck Steak with Smashed Root Veggies

Gluten-Free

SERVES 2 | PREP TIME: 10 MINUTES | COOK TIME: 1 HOUR

Pot roast is my ultimate comfort meal. However, a typical pot roast is huge, which is why I've scaled it down by using chuck steaks instead. Bonus, it takes less time to cook, too!

12 ounces to 1 pound chuck steak

1 teaspoon sea salt, plus more to taste

1 teaspoon freshly ground black pepper

1 tablespoon avocado oil or extra-virgin olive oil

½ white onion, chopped

4 garlic cloves, minced

¼ low-carb dry red wine

¼ cup beef stock

1 large parsnip, peeled and cut into ½-inch pieces

1 large carrot, peeled and cut into ½-inch pieces

1 tablespoon chopped fresh rosemary

1 tablespoon chopped fresh thyme leaves

1 tablespoon butter

1. Preheat the oven to 350°F.

2. Season the chuck steak with the salt and pepper.

3. In a large ovenproof skillet or Dutch oven, heat the oil over medium-high heat. Add the steak and cook for 3 to 5 minutes per side, until it begins to brown. Remove from the skillet and place on a plate.

4. In the same skillet, cook the onion and garlic for 2 to 3 minutes, until the onion begins to brown. Add the red wine and beef stock, scraping up any cooked bits on the bottom of the skillet. Add the parsnip, carrot, rosemary, and thyme. Return the steak to the skillet along with any plate drippings.

5. Cover, transfer to the oven, and bake for 45 minutes to 1 hour, until the steak is tender.

6. Transfer the parsnips and carrots to a medium bowl. Add the butter and smash with a fork. Season with salt and pepper to taste.

7. Divide the steak between two plates and serve with the smashed vegetables on the side. Drizzle with the pan drippings.

DIETARY TIP: For a dish with fewer carbs, swap out the parsnips and carrots for broccoli and cauliflower, but add in the last 20 to 25 minutes of baking instead.

Per serving: Calories: 586; Total fat: 42g; Saturated Fat: 17g; Total Carbs: 20g; Fiber: 5g; Net Carbs: 15g; Protein: 34g; Sodium: 610mg; Sweetener: 0g

Macros: Fat: 64%; Carbs: 13%; Protein: 23%

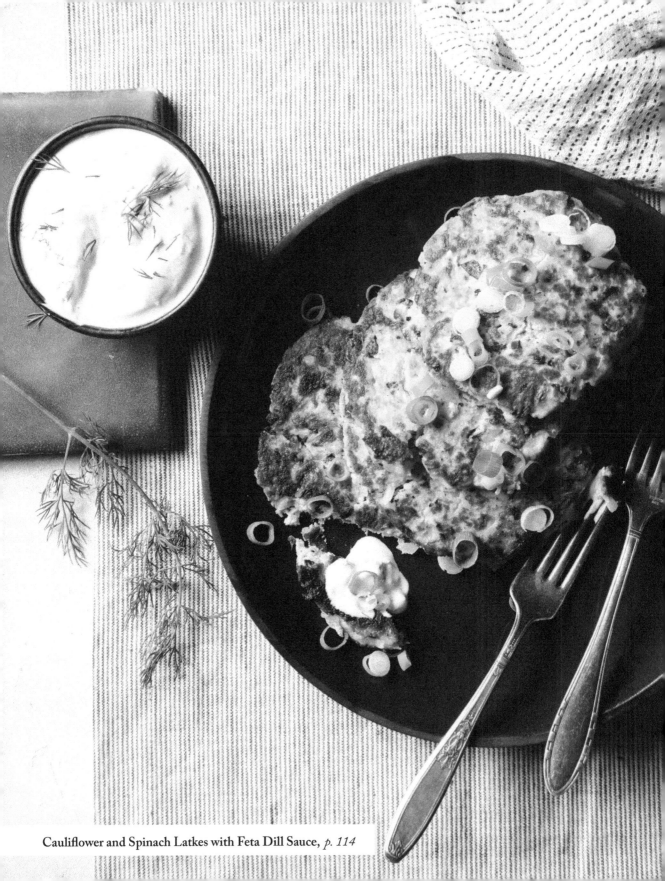

Cauliflower and Spinach Latkes with Feta Dill Sauce, *p. 114*

Fried Green Tomatoes
with Cajun Aioli

Extra Low-Carb, Gluten-Free, Vegetarian

SERVES 2 | PREP TIME: 10 MINUTES | COOK TIME: 15 MINUTES

Summertime in the South always calls for fried green tomatoes. This Southern staple dish can be served as an appetizer, a side, or a vegetarian entrée. When selecting a green tomato, choose a large firm fruit that is uniformly green.

3 tablespoons mayonnaise

1 lemon, ½ juiced and ½ cut into wedges, for serving

2 teaspoons Cajun seasoning

1 garlic clove, minced

½ teaspoon sea salt, plus more to taste

½ teaspoon freshly ground black pepper, plus more to taste

½ cup almond flour

2 tablespoons grated Parmesan cheese

1 teaspoon baking soda

½ teaspoon paprika

1 large egg

¼ cup avocado oil

1 large green tomato, cut into ¼-inch-thick slices

Chopped fresh basil, for garnish

1. In a small bowl, mix together the mayonnaise, lemon juice, Cajun seasoning, and garlic. Season with salt and pepper to taste.

2. Set a wire rack over a baking sheet and set aside.

3. On a large plate, mix together the almond flour, Parmesan, baking soda, paprika, ½ teaspoon salt, and ½ teaspoon pepper. In a small bowl, lightly whisk the egg.

4. In a 10-inch cast-iron skillet, heat the avocado oil over medium-high heat for 1 minute.

5. Working in batches of about 3 slices, dip the tomatoes in the egg, then dredge in the almond flour mixture. Fry for 2 to 3 minutes per side, until golden and crispy. Drain the tomatoes on the rack. Repeat with the remaining tomato slices.

6. Divide the tomato slices between two plates and top with about 2 tablespoons of aioli. Sprinkle with basil and serve with lemon wedges for squeezing.

Per serving: Calories: 461; Total fat: 43g; Saturated Fat: 6g; Total Carbs: 12g; Fiber: 4g; Net Carbs: 8g; Protein: 10g; Sodium: 881mg; Sweetener: 0g

Macros: Fat: 82%; Carbs: 10%; Protein: 8%

Thyme-Roasted Roma Tomatoes

Dairy-Free, Extra Low-Carb, Gluten-Free, Low-Sodium, Vegan

SERVES 2 | PREP TIME: 5 MINUTES | COOK TIME: 35 MINUTES

These tomatoes are like nature's candy! Roasting them brings out their natural sweetness, and the garlic and thyme add a hint of earthiness. This recipe is wonderful served as a side dish, atop a salad, or even eaten as a snack.

4 Roma (plum) tomatoes, cut into ¼-inch-thick slices

6 garlic cloves, chopped

1 tablespoon avocado oil or extra-virgin olive oil

½ teaspoon sea salt

½ teaspoon freshly ground black pepper

5 thyme sprigs, leaves picked

1. Preheat the oven to 450°F. Line a baking sheet with parchment paper.

2. In a medium bowl, combine the tomatoes, garlic, oil, salt, and pepper. Mix well and spread on the prepared baking sheet. Roast for 20 to 30 minutes, until the tomatoes begin to caramelize.

3. Remove from the oven, sprinkle with the thyme leaves, return to the oven, and roast for an additional 5 minutes.

4. Serve warm.

COOKING TIP: When cutting the Roma tomatoes, keep the slices the same size, which will give you a more even cook time and produce a superior end product.

Per serving: Calories: 118; Total fat: 7g; Saturated Fat: 1g; Total Carbs: 13g; Fiber: 3g; Net Carbs: 10g; Protein: 3g; Sodium: 479mg; Sweetener: 0g

Macros: Fat: 55%; Carbs: 39%; Protein: 6%

Chili and Cumin Fried Cauliflower "Rice"

Dairy-Free, Extra Low-Carb, Gluten-Free, Vegan

SERVES 2 | PREP TIME: 10 MINUTES | COOK TIME: 10 MINUTES

This easy low-carb alternative to fried rice pairs well with any entrée. It has become one of my weeknight go-tos, and I'm sure it will become one for you, too. It is also very versatile, and the spice combination can be easily swapped out for others—try ground ginger and curry powder or Cajun seasoning.

1 tablespoon avocado oil or extra-virgin olive oil
½ white onion, minced
3 garlic cloves, chopped
2 cups riced cauliflower

1 tablespoon chili powder
1 teaspoon ground cumin
½ teaspoon sea salt
½ teaspoon freshly ground black pepper

2 tablespoons chopped fresh cilantro, for garnish
1 scallion, chopped
½ lime, juiced

1. In a medium skillet, heat the oil over medium-high heat until shimmering. Add the onion and garlic and stir-fry for 2 minutes, or until the onion starts to soften.

2. Add the riced cauliflower and stir-fry for 5 to 7 minutes, until tender and lightly browned. Add the chili powder, cumin, salt, and pepper. Cook for another 3 minutes, stirring constantly, until the cauliflower is tender.

3. Divide between two plates and garnish with the cilantro, scallions, and lime juice.

COOKING TIP: Be patient and let your skillet and oil heat up, for at least 1 minute. Getting the pan hot will give the onions and garlic a toasty flavor and enhance their natural sweetness.

Per serving: Calories: 125; Total fat: 8g; Saturated Fat: 1g; Total Carbs: 13g; Fiber: 5g; Net Carbs: 8g; Protein: 4g; Sodium: 597mg; Sweetener: 0g

Macros: Fat: 56%; Carbs: 36%; Protein: 8%

Pan-Fried Okra with Creamy Jalapeño Sauce

Gluten-Free, Vegetarian

SERVES 2 | PREP TIME: 15 MINUTES | COOK TIME: 15 MINUTES

My mother-in-law showed me the proper way to prepare okra, and I've loved it ever since. When I went low-carb, I knew that I had to figure out a way to adapt her recipe, and luckily for me—and you—this version tastes just as amazing.

⅓ cup sour cream

1 jalapeño, stemmed and seeded

2 tablespoons chopped fresh cilantro

Juice of 1 lime

1 garlic clove, peeled

2 large eggs

½ cup almond flour

⅓ cup grated Parmesan cheese

½ teaspoon baking powder

½ teaspoon sea salt

½ teaspoon freshly ground black pepper

2 cups ¼-inch slices fresh okra

2 tablespoons avocado oil

1. Set a wire rack on a baking sheet and set aside.

2. In a food processor or blender, blend the sour cream, jalapeño, cilantro, lime juice, and garlic until creamy.

3. In a small bowl, whisk the eggs and set aside. In a large zip-top bag, combine the almond flour, Parmesan, baking powder, salt, and pepper.

4. Add the okra to the egg mixture and then add them to the bag with the almond flour mixture. Seal and shake until the okra is well coated.

5. In a large skillet, heat the avocado oil over medium heat until shimmering. Working in batches, shake the excess flour off the okra and cook for 6 to 8 minutes, until crispy and golden. Flip the okra a couple of times to ensure it does not burn. Remove and place on the wire rack to drain.

6. Divide the okra between two plates with a small bowl of dipping sauce on the side. Serve hot.

DIETARY SWAP: Make this dish vegan by replacing the Parmesan with the same amount of almond flour.

Per serving: Calories: 518; Total fat: 43g; Saturated Fat: 11g; Total Carbs: 19g; Fiber: 7g; Net Carbs: 12g; Protein: 19g; Sodium: 1,075mg; Sweetener: 0g

Macros: Fat: 72%; Carbs: 14%; Protein: 14%

Cauliflower and Spinach Latkes with Feta Dill Sauce

Extra Low-Carb, Gluten-Free, Vegetarian

SERVES 2 | PREP TIME: 10 MINUTES | COOK TIME: 15 MINUTES

A traditional latke is shredded potato, mixed with matzo meal or flour and shallow-fried. It's crispy and savory, but I promise this low-carb, lower-calorie version doesn't skimp on flavor or texture.

2 tablespoons mayonnaise

2 tablespoons sour cream

Juice of ½ lemon

1 tablespoon crumbled feta cheese

4 garlic cloves, minced, divided

1 teaspoon chopped fresh dill

¾ teaspoon sea salt, divided

1¼ teaspoons freshly ground black pepper, divided

1½ cups riced cauliflower

½ cup finely chopped baby spinach

½ white onion, minced

¼ cup shredded mozzarella cheese

1 large egg

2 tablespoons almond flour

1 tablespoon avocado oil

½ scallion, chopped

1. In a small bowl, mix the mayonnaise, sour cream, lemon juice, feta, 1 minced garlic clove, and the dill. Season with ¼ teaspoon of salt and ¼ teaspoon of pepper.

2. In a microwave-safe medium dish, microwave the cauliflower and ⅓ cup water on high for 5 minutes. Let cool for 5 minutes. Drain the cauliflower into a clean kitchen towel and squeeze out the excess water.

3. In a medium bowl, mix the cauliflower, spinach, onion, mozzarella, egg, almond flour, and remaining 3 minced garlic cloves, 1 teaspoon of pepper, and ½ teaspoon of salt. Form into 4 patties.

4. In a large skillet, heat the oil over medium heat. Cook the latkes 4 to 5 minutes per side, until golden brown.

5. Serve 2 patties per person with a small bowl of dipping sauce on the side. Garnish the patties with the scallion and serve hot.

Per serving: Calories: 325; Total fat: 27g; Saturated Fat: 7g; Total Carbs: 12g; Fiber: 3g; Net Carbs: 9g; Protein: 10g; Sodium: 992mg; Sweetener: 0g

Macros: Fat: 75%; Carbs: 13%; Protein: 12%

Elote-Style Skillet Cauliflower

Extra Low-Carb, Gluten-Free, Vegetarian

SERVES 2 | PREP TIME: 15 MINUTES | COOK TIME: 15 MINUTES

I love elote, or grilled Mexican street corn. The sweet corn slathered in a spicy, tangy, and creamy mix of chili powder, mayo, butter, and lime juice is so delicious. Here cauliflower stands in for the corn, but the real star of the show is the fresh cilantro, lime, and vibrant cream sauce. By swapping the corn out for cauliflower, the calories and the carb count are incredibly decreased. This would be a great side dish for a Taco Tuesday dinner.

2 tablespoons sour cream

Juice of ½ lime

1 tablespoon mayonnaise

1 tablespoon chopped fresh cilantro

1 garlic clove, minced

1 teaspoon freshly ground black pepper

½ teaspoon sea salt

¼ teaspoon chipotle powder

1 tablespoon avocado oil or extra-virgin olive oil

1 head cauliflower, cut into ½-inch pieces

1 teaspoon chili powder

½ teaspoon paprika

2 tablespoons crumbled Cotija or feta cheese

1. In a small bowl, mix together the sour cream, lime juice, mayonnaise, cilantro, garlic, pepper, salt, and chipotle powder until well blended. Refrigerate the sauce until ready to use.

2. In a large skillet, heat the oil over medium heat. Add the cauliflower and season with the chili powder and paprika. Cook for 10 to 12 minutes, stirring frequently, until fork-tender and browned.

3. Divide the cauliflower between two plates. Drizzle with the sauce and garnish with the crumbled cheese.

DIETARY SWAP: To make this dish vegan, replace the sour cream with a plant-based yogurt and omit the Cotija.

Per serving: Calories: 201; Total fat: 17g; Saturated Fat: 5g; Total Carbs: 10g; Fiber: 3g; Net Carbs: 7g; Protein: 5g; Sodium: 680mg; Sweetener: 0g

Macros: Fat: 76%; Carbs: 17%; Protein: 7%

Lobster Moc 'n' Cheese

Gluten-Free

SERVES 4 | PREP TIME: 15 MINUTES | COOK TIME: 15 MINUTES

This creamy and decadent side makes enough for four, so if you're entertaining, serve it with a nicely grilled steak and a fresh garden salad for a dinner that will make your guests feel like they're at a high-end steakhouse. I promise they won't miss the high-carb version! But if this is just for the two of you, then you will love the leftovers just as much.

1 head cauliflower, cut into ¼-inch pieces

½ cup water

½ white onion, minced

2 tablespoons butter

4 garlic cloves, chopped

1 medium lobster tail, shell removed and cut into ¼-inch pieces

½ cup half-and-half

4 ounces full-fat cream cheese, cut into chunks, at room temperature

¼ cup shredded Colby Jack cheese

½ teaspoon paprika

½ teaspoon sea salt

½ teaspoon freshly ground black pepper

1 scallion, green tops only, chopped

1. In a medium skillet, combine the cauliflower and water over medium heat. Cover and cook for 5 minutes, or until the cauliflower is al dente. Drain.

2. Increase the heat to medium high. Add the onion, butter, and garlic and cook for 2 minutes, or until the onion becomes tender. Add the lobster and cook for 4 minutes, or until the flesh turns white.

3. Reduce the heat to medium-low. Stir in the half-and-half, cream cheese, Colby Jack, paprika, salt, and pepper. Cover and cook for 5 minutes, or until the cheese is melted and creamy.

4. Garnish with the scallion greens and serve.

VARIATION: This recipe is flexible: swap in shrimp, crab, or bacon in place of the lobster.

Per serving: Calories: 276; Total fat: 22g; Saturated Fat: 13g; Total Carbs: 8g; Fiber: 2g; Net Carbs: 6g; Protein: 13g; Sodium: 585mg; Sweetener: 0g

Macros: Fat: 69%; Carbs: 12%; Protein: 19%

Garlic and Herb Radish Skillet Fries

Extra Low-Carb, Gluten-Free, Vegetarian

SERVES 2 | PREP TIME: 10 MINUTES | COOK TIME: 15 MINUTES

Growing up, skillet fries were on the menu every week, and I really missed them when I started eating low-carb. Thankfully, these crispy radish skillet fries totally scratch that itch—and I haven't looked back since. Serve these radish fries with scrambled or fried eggs for brunch, or with a burger for dinner.

8 ounces
  radishes, quartered
½ cup water
1 white onion, sliced
1 tablespoon avocado oil
  or extra-virgin olive oil,
  plus more for drizzling

4 garlic cloves, chopped
2 teaspoons fresh
  thyme leaves
1 teaspoon chopped
  fresh rosemary
1 teaspoon freshly ground
  black pepper

½ teaspoon sea salt
2 tablespoons shaved
  Parmesan cheese

1. In a medium skillet, combine the radishes and water over medium heat. Cover and cook for 5 minutes, or until al dente. Drain.

2. Increase the heat to medium-high. Add the onion, oil, garlic, thyme, rosemary, pepper, and salt and cook for 7 to 9 minutes, until the radishes are crispy and browned.

3. Divide between two plates and serve hot. Drizzle with some oil and garnish with the Parmesan.

VARIATION: For a Mexican-inspired version, swap out the thyme for 1 teaspoon cumin and 1 teaspoon chili powder. Instead of Parmesan, finish the fries with a squeeze of lime, chopped cilantro, and crumbled Cotija cheese.

Per serving: Calories: 125; Total fat: 9g; Saturated Fat: 2g; Total Carbs: 10g; Fiber: 3g; Net Carbs: 7g; Protein: 3g; Sodium: 602mg; Sweetener: 0g

Macros: Fat: 61%; Carbs: 31%; Protein: 8%

Beef Jalapeño Popper Dip

Extra Low-Carb, Gluten-Free, Low-Sodium

SERVES 4 | PREP TIME: 10 MINUTES | COOK TIME: 40 MINUTES

This dip is classic comfort-food-without-the-carby-guilt! Make it for a small gathering, or double the recipe and take it to your next potluck. This dip pairs well with a snack plate of cut raw vegetables like celery, peppers, cucumbers, and carrots. And if you're making it just for yourselves, any leftover dip will convert to a delicious topping for zoodles.

4 ounces ground beef

½ white onion, minced

3 garlic cloves, chopped

¼ cup shredded Monterey Jack cheese

4 ounces full-fat cream cheese, cut into chunks, at room temperature

2 tablespoons mayonnaise

2 tablespoons sour cream

1 jalapeño, seeded and chopped

½ teaspoon sea salt

½ teaspoon freshly ground black pepper

¼ cup shredded Cheddar cheese

1 scallion, chopped

1. Preheat the oven to 350°F.

2. In an ovenproof medium skillet, cook the ground beef over medium-high heat for 7 to 9 minutes, until browned. Add the onion and garlic and cook for an additional minute. Drain off the excess grease.

3. Reduce the heat to medium-low. Stir in the Monterey Jack, cream cheese, mayonnaise, sour cream, and jalapeño. Cook for 2 minutes, stirring frequently. Season with the salt and pepper.

4. Sprinkle the Cheddar evenly over the top of the dip. Transfer to the oven and bake for 20 to 30 minutes, until the cheese is melted and heated through.

5. Turn the broiler on high and cook until the cheese is browned and bubbling.

6. Garnish with the scallion and serve.

DIETARY SWAP: Reduce the fat in this recipe by replacing the beef with ground chicken or turkey.

Per serving: Calories: 259; Total fat: 22g; Saturated Fat: 10g; Total Carbs: 4g; Fiber: 1g; Net Carbs: 3g; Protein: 12g; Sodium: 491mg; Sweetener: 0g

Macros: Fat: 76%; Carbs: 6%; Protein: 18%

Horseradish Shrimp Dip

Extra Low-Carb, Gluten-Free, Low-Sodium

SERVES 4 | PREP TIME: 15 MINUTES | COOK TIME: 5 MINUTES

When I was growing up, my parents did a lot of entertaining, and I could always count on seeing this dip (one of my favorites) on the table. Easy to prepare, this appetizer will be the star at your next party. Serve it with an assortment of your favorite fresh vegetables and watch it just disappear.

1 tablespoon avocado oil
  or extra-virgin olive oil
8 ounces shrimp, peeled,
  deveined, and cut into
  ¼-inch pieces
¼ white onion, minced
2 garlic cloves, minced
4 ounces full-fat cream
  cheese, cut into chunks, at
  room temperature

Juice of ½ lemon
2 tablespoons mayonnaise
1 tablespoon
  prepared horseradish
1 tablespoon Sugar-Free
  Ketchup (page 143)
1 teaspoon freshly ground
  black pepper

½ teaspoon
  Worcestershire sauce
½ teaspoon sea salt
½ scallion, chopped
Paprika, for garnish

1. In a medium skillet, heat the oil over medium-high heat. Add the shrimp, onion, and garlic and cook for 3 to 5 minutes, until the shrimp are pink and cooked through.

2. Reduce the heat to medium-low. Stir in the cream cheese, lemon juice, mayonnaise, horseradish, ketchup, pepper, Worcestershire, and salt. Stir until creamy.

3. Transfer to a serving bowl and refrigerate for 30 minutes, until cooled.

4. Garnish with the scallion and sprinkle with paprika.

DIETARY SWAP: Cut the sea salt to ¼ teaspoon to make this dip really low-sodium.

Per serving: Calories: 232; Total fat: 17g; Saturated Fat: 6g; Total Carbs: 3g; Fiber: 1g; Net Carbs: 2g; Protein: 13g; Sodium: 471mg; Sweetener: 0g

Macros: Fat: 71%; Carbs: 6%; Protein: 23%

Buffalo Chicken Bites with Buffalo Sauce

Extra Low-Carb, Gluten-Free

SERVES 2 | PREP TIME: 15 MINUTES | COOK TIME: 30 MINUTES

These wings are a fun twist on the original, and they have a place on my game-day menus and my weeknight dinner menus—I can make a full meal of just these bites with a nice big salad. This is one of those recipes I encourage you to make extras of to ensure you have leftovers in the refrigerator.

Nonstick cooking spray
¼ cup mayonnaise
Juice of ½ lemon
3 garlic cloves,
    minced, divided
2 tablespoons hot
    sauce, divided

2 tablespoons crumbled
    blue cheese, divided
1 tablespoon avocado oil
    or extra-virgin olive oil
½ white onion, diced
½ celery stalk, chopped
8 ounces ground chicken

1 large egg
½ teaspoon sea salt
1 teaspoon freshly ground
    black pepper
1 scallion,
    chopped, divided

1. Preheat the oven to 375°F. Mist 8 cups of a mini muffin pan with cooking spray.

2. In a small bowl, mix the mayonnaise, lemon juice, 1 minced garlic clove,
   1 tablespoon of hot sauce, and 1 tablespoon of blue cheese until well combined. Set
   the blue cheese sauce aside.

3. In a medium skillet, heat the oil over medium-high heat for 30 seconds. Add the
   onion, celery, and remaining 2 minced garlic cloves. Cook for 5 minutes, or until the
   onion is tender. Remove from the heat and cool for 5 minutes.

4. Mix in the chicken, egg, salt, pepper, half the scallion, and the remaining
   1 tablespoon of hot sauce and 1 tablespoon of blue cheese. Divide into the
   8 prepared mini muffin cups. Bake for 20 to 25 minutes, until the juices run clear.

5. Serve 4 chicken bites per person, drizzled with the blue cheese sauce and garnished
   with the remaining scallion.

VARIATION: Instead of the Buffalo blue cheese sauce, serve with my Sugar-Free Ranch
Dressing (page 145).

Per serving: Calories: 503; Total fat: 42g; Saturated Fat: 9g; Total Carbs: 6g; Fiber: 1g;
Net Carbs: 5g; Protein: 26g; Sodium: 838mg; Sweetener: 0g

Macros: Fat: 75%; Carbs: 5%; Protein: 20%

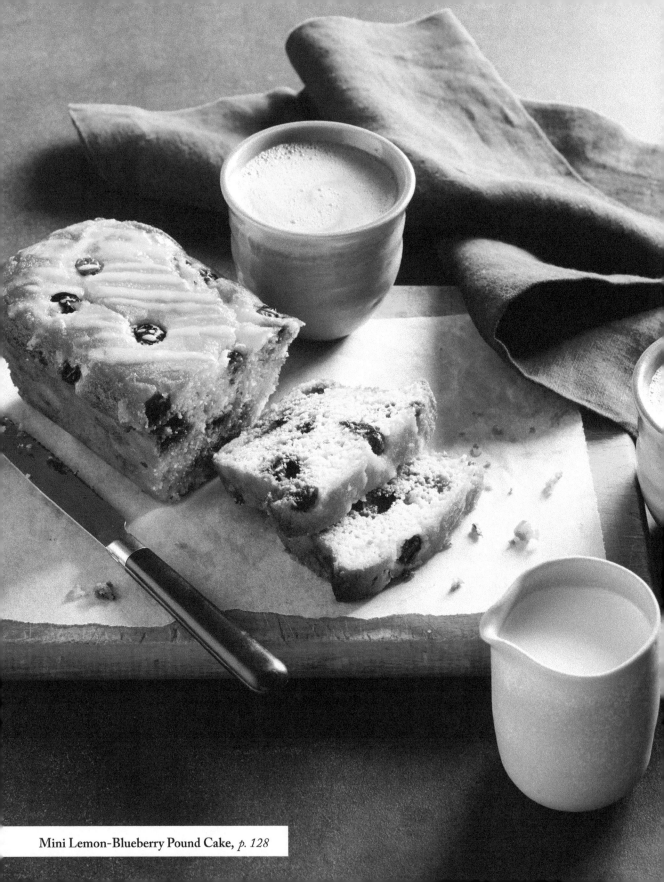

Mini Lemon-Blueberry Pound Cake, *p. 128*

SWEET TREATS

Vanilla Ice Cream

Extra Low-Carb, Gluten-Free, Low-Sodium, Vegetarian

SERVES 2 | PREP TIME: 15 MINUTES, PLUS 1 HOUR TO FREEZE

Who says you can't have ice cream when you're low-carb? This simple three-ingredient ice cream recipe is so rich and creamy that you will always want to have some on hand in your freezer. Top with some sugar-free syrup, fresh berries, or chopped nuts to take care of that sweet tooth. Replacing the heavy cream with coconut cream makes this ice cream vegan, but you may need to whip the coconut cream a bit longer than the dairy cream.

½ cup heavy (whipping) cream

2 tablespoons granulated sugar substitute

1 teaspoon vanilla extract

1. In a medium bowl, with a hand mixer on medium-high, whip the cream, sugar substitute, and vanilla for 1 to 2 minutes, or until soft peaks are formed.

2. Place in an airtight container with a lid and freeze for at least 1 hour.

VARIATIONS: For chocolate peanut butter chip ice cream: Add 1 tablespoon cocoa powder, 1 tablespoon peanut butter, and fold 2 tablespoons sugar-free chocolate chips into the cream mixture. For maple butter pecan: Replace the vanilla with a butter extract and fold in 1 tablespoon chopped pecans and 2 tablespoons sugar-free maple-flavored syrup.

Per serving: Calories: 211; Total fat: 22g; Saturated Fat: 14g; Total Carbs: 2g; Fiber: 0g; Net Carbs: 2g; Protein: 1g; Sodium: 23mg; Sweetener: 12g

Macros: Fat: 93%; Carbs: 4%; Protein: 3%

Cheesecake Mousse Parfaits with Fresh Berries

Extra Low-Carb, Gluten-Free, Low-Sodium, Vegetarian

SERVES 2 | PREP TIME: 10 MINUTES, PLUS 15 MINUTES TO CHILL

This is such a simple, flavorful, and beautiful dessert. Served in parfait glasses or mason jars, the contrast of the white mousse with the red and black berries is stunning. This is an impressive dessert to serve to guests; the ingredients are easily scaled up.

4 ounces full-fat cream cheese, at room temperature

2 tablespoons sour cream

1 tablespoon powdered sugar substitute

Grated zest of 1 lemon

½ teaspoon fresh lemon juice

½ teaspoon vanilla extract

¼ cup heavy (whipping) cream

¼ cup sliced strawberries, plus more for garnish

¼ cup chopped blackberries, plus more for garnish

Fresh mint, for garnish

1. In a medium bowl, with a hand mixer on medium-high, whip the cream cheese, sour cream, powdered sugar substitute, lemon zest, lemon juice, and vanilla for 45 seconds, or until creamy. Add the cream and mix for 1 to 2 minutes, until thick and creamy.

2. In each of two parfait glasses or mason jars, place the strawberries, then ¼ cup mousse, then the blackberries, and top with the remaining ¼ cup of mousse. Refrigerate for at least 15 minutes.

3. Garnish with fresh mint, top with more fresh berries if desired, and serve.

VARIATION: Have fun with the toppings. Sugar-free chocolate chips and chopped toasted nuts are some of my favorites.

Per serving: Calories: 343; Total fat: 33g; Saturated Fat: 19g; Total Carbs: 9g; Fiber: 1g; Net Carbs: 8g; Protein: 5g; Sodium: 225mg; Sweetener: 6g

Macros: Fat: 85%; Carbs: 9%; Protein: 6%

Avocado Key Lime Pudding with Candied Pecans

Extra Low-Carb, Gluten-Free, Low-Sodium, Vegetarian

SERVES 2 | PREP TIME: 10 MINUTES, PLUS 30 MINUTES TO CHILL |
COOK TIME: 5 MINUTES

Avocados are definitely one of the most versatile superfoods out there. They are loaded with healthy fats that are wonderful for the brain and keep you satisfied for a longer period of time. This pudding is so easy to make and is absolutely popping with flavor from the brightness of the lime juice.

2 teaspoons coconut oil

2 tablespoons
  chopped pecans

2 teaspoons brown
  sugar substitute

2 avocados, chilled

¼ cup heavy
  (whipping) cream

Grated zest of
  1 regular lime

Juice of 3 Key limes or
  1 regular lime

½ teaspoon vanilla extract

1. In a small skillet, heat the oil over medium-low heat. Add the pecans and brown sugar substitute and cook, stirring frequently to prevent burning, for 5 minutes, or until the pecans become a shade darker. Set aside to cool for at least 10 minutes.

2. Halve and pit the avocados, then scoop the flesh into a medium bowl. Add the cream, lime zest, lime juice, and vanilla and beat with a hand mixer on medium-high until creamy.

3. Divide the pudding between two juice glasses and refrigerate until chilled, about 30 minutes. Serve topped with the candied pecans.

DIETARY SWAP: Use coconut cream instead of the heavy cream to make this a vegan dessert.

Per serving: Calories: 573; Total fat: 51g; Saturated Fat: 17g; Total Carbs: 31g; Fiber: 18g; Net Carbs: 13g; Protein: 8g; Sodium: 19mg; Sweetener: 4g

Macros: Fat: 76%; Carbs: 19%; Protein: 6%

Chewy Peanut Butter Chocolate Chip Cookies

Extra Low-Carb, Dairy-Free, Gluten-Free, Low-Sodium, Vegetarian

MAKES 6 COOKIES | PREP TIME: 10 MINUTES | COOK TIME: 10 MINUTES

These peanut butter chocolate chip cookies have the texture of an oatmeal cookie without the added carbs from the oats. They are wonderful eaten by themselves or would make the perfect ice cream sandwich with my Vanilla Ice Cream (page 124).

½ cup chunky peanut butter

¼ cup brown sugar substitute

1 large egg

½ teaspoon vanilla extract

⅓ cup almond flour

¼ teaspoon sea salt

¼ teaspoon baking powder

2 tablespoons sugar-free chocolate chips

1. Preheat the oven to 325°F. Line a baking sheet with parchment paper.

2. In a medium bowl, mix the peanut butter, brown sugar substitute, egg, and vanilla until well combined. Add the almond flour, salt, and baking powder and mix until the mixture is creamy. Stir in the chocolate chips.

3. Use a spoon or cookie scoop to divide the mixture into six 2-inch cookies and place on the prepared baking sheet. Bake for 8 to 10 minutes, or until lightly browned and soft.

DIETARY SWAP: Make these cookies vegan by replacing the egg with a flax egg: Mix 1 tablespoon flaxseed with 3 tablespoons water and allow it to sit for 15 minutes before adding to the bowl when you would have added the egg.

Per serving (1 cookie): Calories: 186; Total fat: 15g; Saturated Fat: 3g; Total Carbs: 7g; Fiber: 3g; Net Carbs: 4g; Protein: 7g; Sodium: 94mg; Sweetener: 8g

Macros: Fat: 70%; Carbs: 15%; Protein: 15%

Mini Lemon-Blueberry Pound Cake

Extra Low-Carb, Gluten-Free, Low-Sodium, Vegetarian

SERVES 4 | PREP TIME: 10 MINUTES | COOK TIME: 50 MINUTES

Lemon and blueberry are a match made in sweets heaven. Add cream cheese and you have a moist and decadent pound cake that is bursting with flavor. Enjoy this cake for dessert or with a cup of coffee for an afternoon snack.

Nonstick cooking spray

1 lemon

2 ounces full-fat cream cheese, at room temperature

¼ cup granulated sugar substitute

¼ cup sour cream

1 large egg

1 tablespoon butter, melted

½ teaspoon vanilla extract

½ cup almond flour

½ teaspoon baking powder

¼ cup blueberries

2 tablespoons heavy (whipping) cream

2 tablespoons powdered sugar substitute

1. Preheat the oven to 350°F. Mist a mini loaf pan with cooking spray.

2. Grate the zest from the whole lemon. Juice half the lemon (save the other half for another use) and set the juice aside.

3. In a medium bowl, whisk together the cream cheese, granulated sugar substitute, sour cream, egg, melted butter, and vanilla until well combined. Add the almond flour, baking powder, and lemon zest and mix until well incorporated. Fold in the blueberries. Scrape the batter into the prepared pan.

4. Bake for 40 to 50 minutes, until a toothpick inserted in the center comes out clean.

5. Meanwhile, in a small bowl, combine the cream, powdered sugar substitute, and reserved lemon juice. Whisk the lemon glaze until smooth.

6. Remove the cake from the oven and use a wooden skewer or toothpick to poke numerous holes in the cake. Pour the lemon glaze onto the cake so it drips down into the holes and saturates the cake.

7. Cut into 4 slices and serve.

COOKING TIP: Don't be shy about poking holes in the cake, and make sure you poke all the way through so the glaze soaks the cake evenly.

Per serving (1 slice): Calories: 224; Total fat: 21g; Saturated Fat: 9g; Total Carbs: 6g; Fiber: 2g; Net Carbs: 4g; Protein: 6g; Sodium: 148mg; Sweetener: 18g

Macros: Fat: 80%; Carbs: 10%; Protein: 10%

Double Fudge Brownies

Dairy-Free, Extra Low-Carb, Gluten-Free, Low-Sodium, Vegetarian

SERVES 4 | PREP TIME: 5 MINUTES | COOK TIME: 50 MINUTES

You can never go wrong with double fudge brownies. If you're looking for a fantastic low-carb brownie recipe, this is it. Using cocoa powder in place of melted chocolate helps create a very rich, chewy, and fudgy brownie. These are great eaten alone or topped with homemade whipped cream.

Nonstick cooking spray

¼ cup granulated
  sugar substitute

1 large egg

2 tablespoons avocado oil

½ teaspoon vanilla extract

½ cup almond flour

¼ cup unsweetened
  cocoa powder

¼ teaspoon baking powder

2 tablespoons sugar-free
  chocolate chips

1. Preheat the oven to 350°F. Mist a mini loaf pan with cooking spray.

2. In a medium bowl, mix together the sugar substitute, egg, oil, and vanilla until well blended. Mix in the almond flour, cocoa powder, and baking powder. Stir in the chocolate chips.

3. Bake for 40 to 50 minutes, until a toothpick inserted into the center comes out clean.

4. Cut into 4 slices and serve warm.

VARIATION: Feel free to throw in some chopped pecans or walnuts.

Per serving (1 slice): Calories: 185; Total fat: 18g; Saturated Fat: 3g; Total Carbs: 7g; Fiber: 4g; Net Carbs: 3g; Protein: 6g; Sodium: 44mg; Sweetener: 12g

Macros: Fat: 78%; Carbs: 11%; Protein: 11%

Sea Salt Orange Chocolate Bark

Dairy-Free, Extra Low-Carb, Gluten-Free, Vegan

SERVES 8 | PREP TIME: 10 MINUTES | COOK TIME: 5 MINUTES

This is probably one of the easiest desserts you'll ever make, and you'll be completely surprised by the amazing flavor it offers. The sweetness from the chocolate and the hit of citrus from the orange zest complement the earthiness of the nuts. Bringing it all together is the sea salt on the top. Because the chocolate bark keeps well, this recipe makes enough for multiple treats. Store it in the refrigerator for when the mood strikes.

2 cups sugar-free chocolate chips

1 tablespoon no-sugar-added nut butter of choice

1 tablespoon chopped walnuts

1 tablespoon chopped almonds

1 tablespoon chopped peanuts

Grated zest of ½ orange

½ teaspoon orange extract

2 teaspoons coarse sea salt

1. Line a small baking sheet with parchment paper.

2. In a double boiler or in a glass bowl over a saucepan of simmering water, heat the chocolate and nut butter over medium heat, stirring constantly, for about 5 minutes, or until melted and creamy.

3. Stir in the walnuts, almonds, peanuts, orange zest, and orange extract. Pour onto the prepared baking sheet and use a spatula to spread the mixture into a ¼-inch-thick layer. Sprinkle with the sea salt and refrigerate for 20 minutes.

4. Break into 2-inch pieces and enjoy.

COOKING TIP: When melting the chocolate, make sure no water gets into the bowl, or it will cause your chocolate mixture to seize up.

Per serving: Calories: 363; Total fat: 30g; Saturated Fat: 17g; Total Carbs: 2g; Fiber: 1g; Net Carbs: 1g; Protein: 4g; Sodium: 881mg; Sweetener: 19g

Macros: Fat: 86%; Carbs: 4%; Protein: 10%

Carrot Mug Cakes with Cream Cheese Frosting

Extra Low-Carb, Gluten-Free, Vegetarian

SERVES 2 | PREP TIME: 10 MINUTES, PLUS 10 MINUTES TO COOL |
COOK TIME: 1 MINUTE

Carrot cake is my ultimate favorite and I eat it on every birthday. Here's a quick sized-down low-carb version of the traditional carrot cake. Using freshly shredded carrots and chopped walnuts is the key to make this an over-the-top carrot cake.

Nonstick cooking spray

¼ cup brown
  sugar substitute

1 large egg

1 tablespoon avocado oil

¼ teaspoon vanilla extract

½ cup almond flour

⅓ cup finely
  shredded carrots

½ teaspoon
  ground cinnamon

¼ teaspoon baking powder

¼ teaspoon
  ground nutmeg

¼ teaspoon sea salt

2 tablespoons
  chopped walnuts

4 ounces full-fat
  cream cheese, at
  room temperature

1 tablespoon powdered
  sugar substitute

1. Mist 2 microwave-safe mugs with cooking spray.

2. In a medium bowl, combine the brown sugar substitute, egg, avocado oil, and vanilla until well combined. Mix in the almond flour, carrots, cinnamon, baking powder, nutmeg, and salt. Fold in the walnuts.

3. Divide the batter between the mugs and cook for 45 to 60 seconds, depending on the microwave wattage, until a toothpick inserted in the center comes out clean. Cool for 10 minutes.

4. In a small bowl, stir together the cream cheese and powdered sugar substitute until creamy.

5. Divide the frosting evenly between the cakes and enjoy!

COOKING TIP: For consistency in cooking this quick dessert, it's important to use a small shred for the carrots.

Per serving: Calories: 435; Total fat: 40g; Saturated Fat: 13g; Total Carbs: 9g; Fiber: 3g; Net Carbs: 6g; Protein: 11g; Sodium: 652mg; Sweetener: 30g

Macros: Fat: 82%; Carbs: 8%; Protein: 10%

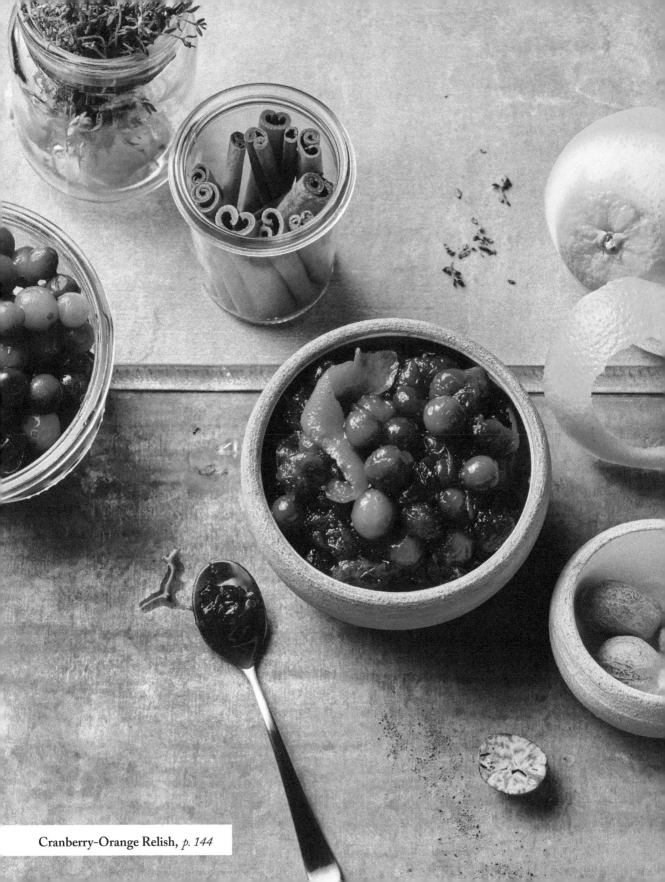

Cranberry-Orange Relish, *p. 144*

Chapter Nine

STAPLES, SAUCES, AND DRESSINGS

Soft and Fluffy Sandwich Bread

Dairy-Free, Extra Low-Carb, Gluten-Free, Low-Sodium, Vegetarian

MAKES 2 "SLICES" | PREP TIME: 10 MINUTES | COOK TIME: 2 MINUTES

This super-easy low-carb bread is soft and pillowy, and reminds me of the classic white bread. It is best made in a mini waffle iron because the steam helps create a softer bread, but you can also cook it up in a skillet. Use this bread to make French toast, open-faced sandwiches, garlic bread, or as burger buns—the possibilities are endless!

1 large egg

1 tablespoon mayonnaise

3 tablespoons almond flour

¼ teaspoon baking powder

⅛ teaspoon sea salt

1. Preheat a mini waffle iron according to manufacturer's instructions. (Alternatively, warm a skillet over low heat.)

2. In a small bowl, mix the egg and mayonnaise. Add the almond flour, baking powder, and salt.

3. Scoop half the batter into the waffle iron and cook according to the manufacturer's instructions. (In the skillet, cook 2 to 3 minutes per side, until firm.) Repeat to make a second "slice."

4. Serve immediately or if making ahead, refrigerate for up to 3 days, or freeze for up to 1 month.

VARIATIONS: This recipe is like a blank canvas. For a delightful garlic and herb bread, add ½ teaspoon garlic powder, ¼ teaspoon minced fresh rosemary, and ¼ teaspoon minced fresh oregano. Or for a sweet version, add ½ teaspoon ground cinnamon and ½ teaspoon brown sugar substitute.

Per serving (1 "slice"): Calories: 138; Total fat: 12g; Saturated Fat: 2g; Total Carbs: 2g; Fiber: 1g; Net Carbs: 1g; Protein: 5g; Sodium: 204mg; Sweetener: 0g

Macros: Fat: 78%; Carbs: 7%; Protein: 15%

"Fathead" Pizza Crust

Extra Low-Carb, Gluten-Free, Low-Sodium, Vegetarian

SERVES 2 | PREP TIME: 10 MINUTES | COOK TIME: 17 MINUTES

This simple pizza crust recipe has been popular in low-carb circles for quite some time. It's super versatile, so try using it to make a calzone or flatbread. Get creative!

1½ cups shredded
   mozzarella cheese

2 tablespoons full-fat
   cream cheese
¾ cup almond flour

1 large egg
½ teaspoon sea salt

1. Preheat the oven to 425°F. Line a baking sheet with parchment paper.

2. In a microwave-safe bowl, heat the mozzarella and cream cheese in the microwave in 30-second intervals, until the cheese is melted. Let cool for 2 minutes.

3. Mix in the almond flour, egg, and salt.

4. Transfer the dough to the prepared baking sheet and form into a ¼-inch-thick round. Prick the dough with a fork about 12 times to prevent bubbling.

5. Bake for 8 minutes. Prick any air bubbles and bake for an additional 7 minutes, or until browned.

6. Add toppings of choice and bake to heat the toppings and melt any cheese you've used.

COOKING TIPS: It's very important to prick the dough with a fork to prevent large air bubbles from forming in the crust. Also keep in mind that any ingredients you put on top of this crust need to be precooked, as the crust goes back into the oven just long enough to heat things through.

Per serving: Calories: 544; Total fat: 42g; Saturated Fat: 16g; Total Carbs: 10g; Fiber: 4g; Net Carbs: 6g; Protein: 30g; Sodium: 906mg; Sweetener: 0g

Macros: Fat: 69%; Carbs: 9%; Protein: 22%

Shredded Cabbage Noodles

Dairy-Free, Extra Low-Carb, Gluten-Free, Low-Sodium, Vegan

MAKES 2 CUPS | PREP TIME: 5 MINUTES | COOK TIME: 10 MINUTES

You may have had zucchini noodles ("zoodles"), but have you tried cabbage noodles? These savory cabbage noodles are light, low-carb, and the perfect substitute for noodles in a flavorful lo mein or for pasta topped with my Classic Marinara Sauce (page 142).

2 tablespoons avocado oil or extra-virgin olive oil

1 head cabbage, cut into ¼-inch-wide shreds

½ white onion, thinly sliced

4 garlic cloves, chopped

Sea salt

Freshly ground black pepper

1. In a large skillet, heat the oil over medium-high heat for 30 seconds.

2. Add the cabbage, onion, and garlic and cook for 7 to 9 minutes, until the cabbage is firm-tender. Season with salt and pepper to taste and serve hot.

COOKING TIP: When prepping the cabbage, cut the core out first for more even shreds.

Per serving: Calories: 229; Total fat: 14g; Saturated Fat: 2g; Total Carbs: 24g; Fiber: 9g; Net Carbs: 15g; Protein: 5g; Sodium: 143mg; Sweetener: 0g

Macros: Fat: 55%; Carbs: 39%; Protein: 6%

Mashed Cauliflower and Root Medley

Gluten-Free, Low-Sodium, Vegetarian

MAKES 2½ CUPS | PREP TIME: 15 MINUTES | COOK TIME: 20 MINUTES

This healthy mashed root medley will quickly replace your carb-loaded mashed potatoes. Serve it alongside a grilled steak, grilled chicken, or grilled pork. It also goes well with a Thanksgiving Day feast along with my Cranberry-Orange Relish (page 144).

1 small carrot, peeled and cut into ¼-inch pieces
1 small parsnip, peeled and cut into ¼-inch pieces
½ small head cauliflower, cut into florets
1 cup half-and-half
2 ounces full-fat cream cheese, cut into chunks, at room temperature
2 tablespoons butter
4 garlic cloves, minced
3 thyme sprigs, leaves picked
¼ teaspoon ground nutmeg
Sea salt
Freshly ground black pepper
1 tablespoon chopped fresh chives

1. In a saucepan, combine the carrot, parsnip, and cauliflower. Add cold water to cover by 2 inches. Bring to a boil over medium-high heat, then reduce the temperature to medium and simmer for 10 to 15 minutes, until the vegetables are tender. Drain and return to the pan.

2. Add the half-and-half, cream cheese, butter, and garlic. Cover and let sit for 5 minutes.

3. Using a hand mixer, blend until smooth and creamy. Add the thyme leaves and nutmeg. Season with salt and pepper to taste.

4. Serve immediately, garnished with chives.

DIETARY SWAP: For a vegan option, omit the butter, half-and-half, and cream cheese. Instead of blending the vegetables until smooth, drizzle them with olive oil and smash until chunky.

Per serving (½ cup): Calories: 178; Total fat: 14g; Saturated Fat: 9g; Total Carbs: 11g; Fiber: 3g; Net Carbs: 8g; Protein: 3g; Sodium: 117mg; Sweetener: 0g

Macros: Fat: 70%; Carbs: 23%; Protein: 7%

Nashville Hot Chicken Seasoning

Dairy-Free, Extra Low-Carb, Gluten-Free, Low-Sodium, Vegan

MAKES ¼ CUP | PREP TIME: 5 MINUTES | COOK TIME: 20 MINUTES

If you have not tried Nashville hot chicken, you are totally missing out. This seasoning offers a balanced sweet and spicy flavor profile and will keep you coming back for more. Of course, it's great on chicken, but I also like to sauté cauliflower in this seasoning. Store in an airtight container in a cool, dark place for up to 6 months.

3 tablespoons cayenne pepper

1 tablespoon brown sugar substitute

1 teaspoon garlic powder

1 teaspoon paprika

½ teaspoon chili powder

½ teaspoon salt

In a small bowl, combine the cayenne, brown sugar substitute, garlic powder, paprika, chili powder, and salt. Mix and enjoy.

VARIATION: To turn down the heat, omit the cayenne and replace it with 1 tablespoon ground white pepper.

Per serving (1 teaspoon): Calories: 6; Total fat: 0g; Saturated Fat: 0g; Total Carbs: 5g; Fiber: 0g; Net Carbs: 1g; Protein: 0g; Sodium: 101mg; Sweetener: 4g

Macros: Fat: 38%; Carbs: 48%; Protein: 14%

Italian Seasoning

Dairy-Free, Extra Low-Carb, Gluten-Free, Low-Sodium, Vegan

MAKES ¼ CUP | PREP TIME: 5 MINUTES | COOK TIME: 20 MINUTES

This Italian seasoning is what makes my Homemade Italian Sausage with Red Wine and Tomato Sauce (page 97) tick. It's also great on beef and pork, in spaghetti sauce, and with all things Italian. Or use as a seasoning base for a vinaigrette dressing. Store in an airtight container in a cool, dark place for up to 6 months.

1 tablespoon fennel seeds
½ tablespoon
   dried oregano
½ tablespoon dried basil
½ tablespoon
   onion powder

½ tablespoon
   garlic powder
½ tablespoon dried parsley
½ teaspoon red
   pepper flakes

½ teaspoon sea salt
¼ teaspoon freshly ground
   black pepper

In a small bowl, mix the fennel seeds, oregano, basil, onion powder, garlic powder, parsley, red pepper flakes, salt, and black pepper.

COOKING TIP: For an easy and soul-satisfying meat sauce, season 8 ounces ground beef with 1 tablespoon of the seasoning and brown, then add my Classic Marinara Sauce (page 142).

Per serving (1 teaspoon): Calories: 4; Total fat: 0g; Saturated Fat: 0g; Total Carbs: 1g; Fiber: 0g; Net Carbs: 1g; Protein: 0g; Sodium: 49mg; Sweetener: 0g

Macros: Fat: 16%; Carbs: 71%; Protein: 13%

Classic Marinara Sauce

Dairy-Free, Gluten-Free, Vegan

MAKES 1½ CUPS | PREP TIME: 5 MINUTES | COOK TIME: 20 MINUTES

There's really no need to pay for expensive store-bought jarred sauces, and with a home-made sauce you can control the added sugars. With so few ingredients, this traditional classic marinara can be on the table in no time, so it's perfect for a busy weeknight meal. It is sure to be your new go-to recipe for Italian-inspired meals.

½ white onion, minced

2 tablespoons extra-virgin olive oil

4 garlic cloves, minced

1 (14.5-ounce) can crushed tomatoes

1 teaspoon freshly ground black pepper

½ teaspoon sea salt

¼ teaspoon red pepper flakes

¼ cup chopped fresh basil

1. In a saucepan, combine the onion, oil, and garlic over medium heat. Cook for 4 minutes, or until the onions become tender.

2. Reduce the heat to medium-low. Add the crushed tomatoes, black pepper, salt, and red pepper flakes and simmer for 15 minutes to meld the flavors.

3. Stir in the basil and serve.

VARIATION: Add ¼ cup pureed roasted red peppers and ¼ cup heavy (whipping) cream for a richer flavor.

Per serving (½ cup): Calories: 145; Total fat: 9g; Saturated Fat: 1g; Total Carbs: 15g; Fiber: 3g; Net Carbs: 12g; Protein: 3g; Sodium: 621mg; Sweetener: 0g

Macros: Fat: 57%; Carbs: 38%; Protein: 5%

Sugar-Free Ketchup

Dairy-Free, Extra Low-Carb, Gluten-Free, Low-Sodium, Vegan

MAKES 2¼ CUPS | PREP TIME: 5 MINUTES | COOK TIME: 5 MINUTES

The majority of store-bought ketchups are loaded with sugar. Here's a simple recipe that will scratch the ketchup itch without all the carbs. Bonus: This recipe works as a base for other sauces (see Variations, below).

1 cup water

6 ounces tomato paste

¼ cup brown
   sugar substitute

¼ cup distilled
   white vinegar

1 teaspoon sea salt

1 teaspoon onion powder

1 teaspoon garlic powder

1 teaspoon smoked paprika

⅛ teaspoon ground cloves

In a saucepan, whisk together the water, tomato paste, brown sugar substitute, vinegar, salt, onion powder, garlic powder, smoked paprika, and ground cloves over medium-low heat. Simmer for 5 minutes, stirring frequently to prevent the sauce from sticking to the sides of the saucepan.

VARIATIONS: For a barbecue sauce: Add 1 teaspoon liquid smoke, 1 teaspoon soy sauce, and 1 teaspoon Worcestershire sauce. For a sweet and sour sauce: Combine ¼ cup of the ketchup, ½ cup apple cider vinegar, ¼ cup brown sugar substitute, 2 tablespoons soy sauce, 1 teaspoon garlic powder, 1 teaspoon ground ginger, and ½ teaspoon sesame oil.

Per serving (2 tablespoons): Calories: 10; Total fat: 0g; Saturated Fat: 0g; Total Carbs: 5g; Fiber: 1g; Net Carbs: 1g; Protein: 0g; Sodium: 103mg; Sweetener: 3g

Macros: Fat: 6%; Carbs: 81%; Protein: 13%

Cranberry-Orange Relish

Dairy-Free, Extra Low-Carb, Gluten-Free, Low-Sodium, Vegan

MAKES ABOUT 1 CUP | PREP TIME: 5 MINUTES | COOK TIME: 20 MINUTES

This is the cranberry-orange relish my father taught me to make decades ago, and when I went low-carb, I transformed it so I could still make it every Thanksgiving, guilt-free. But don't feel like you're limited to only having this on Thanksgiving! It makes a nice spread for a turkey sandwich, as a topping for Greek yogurt, or in place of the berry layers in my Cheesecake Mousse Parfaits with Fresh Berries (page 125).

6 ounces fresh cranberries

1 cup water

¼ cup brown
   sugar substitute

Grated zest and juice of
   1 orange

1 cinnamon stick

½ teaspoon
   ground nutmeg

2 thyme sprigs,
   leaves picked

In a medium saucepan, combine the cranberries, water, brown sugar substitute, orange zest, orange juice, cinnamon stick, nutmeg, and thyme leaves. Bring to a simmer over medium-low heat and cook for 15 to 25 minutes, until the sauce reduces by one-quarter and begins to thicken. Refrigerate until ready to serve.

COOKING TIP: The key to this sauce is a slow and steady simmer, which produces a thick cranberry relish.

Per serving (¼ cup): Calories: 31; Total fat: 0g; Saturated Fat: 0g; Total Carbs: 20g; Fiber: 2g; Net Carbs: 6g; Protein: 0g; Sodium: 1mg; Sweetener: 12g

Macros: Fat: 5%; Carbs: 91%; Protein: 4%

Sugar-Free Ranch Dressing

Extra Low-Carb, Gluten-Free, Low-Sodium, Vegetarian

MAKES ABOUT 1¼ CUPS | PREP TIME: 10 MINUTES

Ranch dressing is a staple in my kitchen, but store-bought versions usually have sugar. I knew I had to make this dressing low-carb when I started this lifestyle. This dressing conveniently serves as a base for many other recipes: Try out some of the suggested variations that follow, or experiment and make your own.

½ cup mayonnaise

½ cup sour cream

2 tablespoons half-and-half

1 teaspoon dried dill weed

½ teaspoon dried parsley

½ teaspoon onion powder

½ teaspoon garlic powder

½ teaspoon dried chives

Juice of ½ lemon

½ teaspoon sea salt

½ teaspoon freshly ground black pepper

In a medium bowl, mix together the mayonnaise, sour cream, half-and-half, dill, parsley, onion powder, garlic powder, chives, lemon juice, salt, and pepper until well combined. Store in the refrigerator until ready to use.

VARIATIONS: For jalapeño ranch: Swap the dill for cilantro and add ½ a minced jalapeño. For cracked pepper and Parmesan ranch: Add an additional 1½ teaspoons freshly ground black pepper and 1 tablespoon grated Parmesan. For chipotle ranch: Add 2 teaspoons chipotle powder and swap the lemon juice for lime.

Per serving (2 tablespoons): Calories: 103; Total fat: 11g; Saturated Fat: 3g; Total Carbs: 1g; Fiber: 0g; Net Carbs: 1g; Protein: 1g; Sodium: 147mg; Sweetener: 0g

Macros: Fat: 95%; Carbs: 3%; Protein: 2%

Sugar-Free Honey Mustard

Dairy-Free, Extra Low-Carb, Gluten-Free, Low-Sodium, Vegetarian

MAKES ¾ CUP | PREP TIME: 10 MINUTES | COOK TIME: 1 MINUTE

Honey mustard is one of my favorite dressings. I just love the sweetness with a touch of spice. This low-carb version is perfect for marinating chicken or pork, used as a dip for my Paprika Fish Sticks with Rémoulade Sauce (page 84) instead of the rémoulade, or drizzled on a large fresh garden salad.

3 tablespoons brown
  sugar substitute
1 teaspoon water

½ cup mayonnaise
¼ cup Dijon mustard

⅛ teaspoon
  smoked paprika

1. In a microwave-safe bowl, combine the brown sugar substitute and water and microwave on high for 30 seconds, until the sugar is dissolved. Cool for 5 minutes.

2. Add the mayonnaise, mustard, and smoked paprika and mix until well blended.

3. Serve as a salad dressing or as a dipping sauce. Store leftovers in an airtight container in the refrigerator for up to 1 week.

DIETARY SWAP: To reduce the sodium, replace the Dijon mustard with 1 tablespoon mustard powder and 1 teaspoon apple cider vinegar.

Per serving (2 tablespoons): Calories: 131; Total fat: 14g; Saturated Fat: 3g; Total Carbs: 7g; Fiber: 0g; Net Carbs: 1g; Protein: 1g; Sodium: 231mg; Sweetener: 6g

Macros: Fat: 96%; Carbs: 2%; Protein: 2%

Raspberry Balsamic Vinaigrette

Dairy-Free, Extra Low-Carb, Gluten-Free, Low-Sodium, Vegan

MAKES ½ CUP | PREP TIME: 10 MINUTES | COOK TIME: 1 MINUTE

This sweet and tart vinaigrette is one I like to have on hand for my leafy green salads. I also like to use it as a marinade for firm white fish, chicken, or pork—the bold flavors from the balsamic and Dijon complement these proteins quite nicely.

10 fresh raspberries

1 tablespoon water

¼ cup avocado oil or extra-virgin olive oil

2 tablespoons balsamic vinegar

Juice of ½ lemon

1 garlic clove, minced

1 teaspoon granulated sugar substitute

½ teaspoon Dijon mustard

Sea salt

Freshly ground black pepper

1. In a microwave-safe bowl, combine the raspberries and water. Microwave on high for 30 seconds. Using the back of a spoon, mash the berries. Cool for 5 minutes.

2. In a screw-top jar, combine the raspberries, oil, balsamic vinegar, lemon juice, garlic, sugar substitute, and mustard. Shake until emulsified. Season with salt and pepper to taste.

COOKING TIP: Don't be afraid to shake that jar HARD. Vigorously shaking will help emulsify the oil in the vinegar to create a creamier vinaigrette.

Per serving (2 tablespoons): Calories: 133; Total fat: 14g; Saturated Fat: 2g; Total Carbs: 4g; Fiber: 0g; Net Carbs: 3g; Protein: 0g; Sodium: 48mg; Sweetener: 1g

Macros: Fat: 88%; Carbs: 12%; Protein: 0%

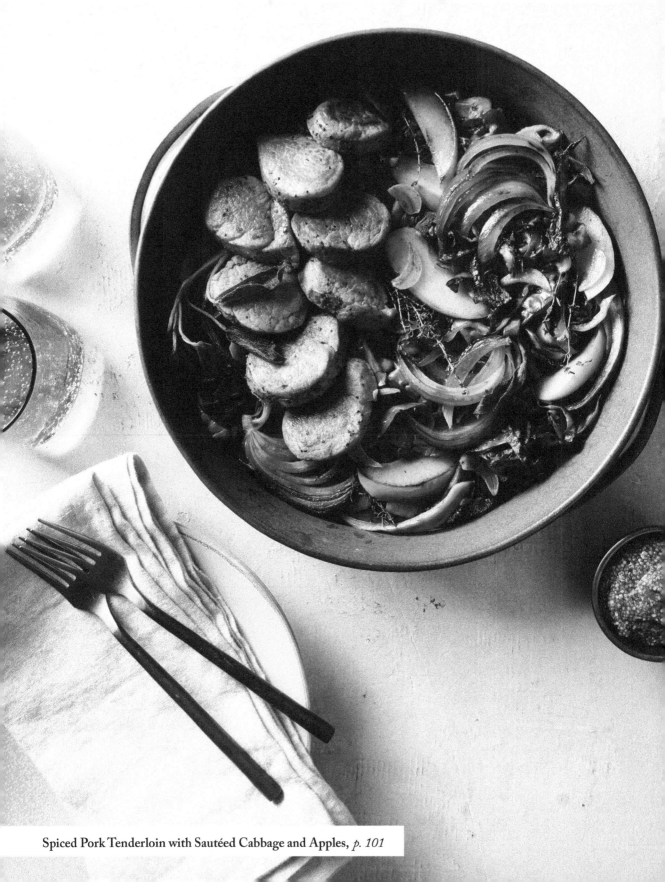

Spiced Pork Tenderloin with Sautéed Cabbage and Apples, *p. 101*

MEASUREMENT CONVERSIONS

VOLUME EQUIVALENTS	U.S. STANDARD	U.S. STANDARD (OUNCES)	METRIC (APPROXIMATE)
LIQUID	2 tablespoons	1 fl. oz.	30 mL
	¼ cup	2 fl. oz.	60 mL
	½ cup	4 fl. oz.	120 mL
	1 cup	8 fl. oz.	240 mL
	1½ cups	12 fl. oz.	355 mL
	2 cups or 1 pint	16 fl. oz.	475 mL
	4 cups or 1 quart	32 fl. oz.	1 L
	1 gallon	128 fl. oz.	4 L
DRY	⅛ teaspoon	–	0.5 mL
	¼ teaspoon	–	1 mL
	½ teaspoon	–	2 mL
	¾ teaspoon	–	4 mL
	1 teaspoon	–	5 mL
	1 tablespoon	–	15 mL
	¼ cup	–	59 mL
	⅓ cup	–	79 mL
	½ cup	–	118 mL
	⅔ cup	–	156 mL
	¾ cup	–	177 mL
	1 cup	–	235 mL
	2 cups or 1 pint	–	475 mL
	3 cups	–	700 mL
	4 cups or 1 quart	–	1 L
	½ gallon	–	2 L
	1 gallon	–	4 L

OVEN TEMPERATURES

FAHRENHEIT	CELSIUS (APPROXIMATE)
250°F	120°C
300°F	150°C
325°F	165°C
350°F	180°C
375°F	190°C
400°F	200°C
425°F	220°C
450°F	230°C

WEIGHT EQUIVALENTS

U.S. STANDARD	METRIC (APPROXIMATE)
½ ounce	15 g
1 ounce	30 g
2 ounces	60 g
4 ounces	115 g
8 ounces	225 g
12 ounces	340 g
16 ounces or 1 pound	455 g

RESOURCES

Informational Websites

Diet Doctor:
DietDoctor.com

Ditch the Carbs:
DitchTheCarbs.com

Low-Carb Practitioners:
LowCarbPractitioners.com

Low Carb USA:
LowCarbUSA.org

Books

Bowden, Jonny. *Living Low Carb: Controlled-Carbohydrate Eating for Long-Term Weight Loss*. New York: Sterling Publishing, 2013.

Lustig, Robert H. *Fat Change: Beating the Odds Against Sugar, Processed Food, Obesity, and Disease*. New York: Avery, 2013.

Volek, Jeff S. and Stephen D. Phinney. *The Art and Science of Low Carbohydrate Living: An Expert Guide to Making the Life-Saving Benefits of Carbohydrate Restriction Sustainable and Enjoyable*. Self-published: 2011.

Tracking Apps

Carb Manager App
(CarbManager.com)

CronOMeter
(CronoMeter.com)

My Fitness Pal
(MyFitnessPal.com)

Online Shopping

Porter Road Butcher: This online butcher sells pasture-raised meats with no antibiotics or added hormones.
PorterRoad.com

Secco Wine: Keto, Paleo, and Low-Carb Italian wines.
SeccoWine.com

Sizzle Fish: An online seafood market with lobster, salmon, shrimp, scallops, cod, and more.
Sizzlefish.com

REFERENCES

Diabetes Forecast. "How the Body Uses Carbohydrates, Proteins, and Fats." Accessed on June 1, 2020. http://www.diabetesforecast.org/2011/mar/how-the-body-uses-carbohydrates-proteins-and-fats.html

Harvard T.H. Chan School of Public Health. "Diabetes." Accessed on June 1, 2020. https://www.hsph.harvard.edu/nutritionsource/disease-prevention/diabetes-prevention/

Harvard T.H. Chan School of Public Health. "Low-Carb Diets." Accessed on June 1, 2020. https://www.hsph.harvard.edu/nutritionsource/carbohydrates/low-carbohydrate-diets/

Stanford Medical School. "Higher percentages of saturated fat in the low-carb diets may not harm cholesterol levels, new analysis finds." Accessed on June 1, 2020. https://scopeblog.stanford.edu/2019/01/16/higher-percentages-of-saturated-fat-in-low-carb-diets-may-not-harm-cholesterol-levels-new-analysis-suggests/

INDEX

ACKNOWLEDGMENTS

Randy, thanks for always closing the refrigerator for me.

Cade and Caitlyn, thank you for being my on-call taste testers.

To my family and friends, thank you for your constant support, encouragement, and all the recipe brainstorming sessions.

To my online community, thank you for keeping me motivated to be the best. I am beyond grateful for each of you.

ABOUT THE AUTHOR

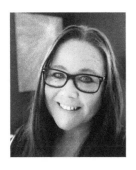

Bek Davis is a trained chef and recipe developer and has been in the food industry since she was 16 years old. Bek started living a low-carb lifestyle in 2015 in order to shed excess weight. Luckily, Bek's culinary arts background gave her the knowledge to transform high-carb dishes into low-carb versions with ease. As Bek started to lose weight, her friends and family wanted in on her low-carb recipes. She decided to start posting her recipes online—and the rest is history!

Bek resides with her husband just outside of Nashville, Tennessee, and often escapes to her Chattanooga home to spend time with her two college-aged children. Find more of Bek's recipes at lowcarbbek.com or follow her on Instagram (@lowcarbbek).

CPSIA information can be obtained
at www.ICGtesting.com
Printed in the USA
JSHW010716270721
17186JS00005B/7